GROW YOUR OWN

HRT

Sprout Hormone-Rich Greens
in Only Two Minutes a Day

GROW YOUR OWN

HRT

Sprout Hormone-Rich Greens in Only Two Minutes a Day

Sally J. Duffell

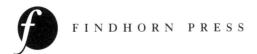

FINDHORN PRESS

Published in 2017 by Findhorn Press, Scotland

ISBN 978-1-84409-737-1

All photos including cover photo by Bea Lacey, *www.laceyfineart.com*

Edited by Nicky Leach
Cover design by Richard Crookes
Interior design by Damian Keenan
Printed and bound in the EU

DISCLAIMER

The information in this book (in print and electronic media)
is given in good faith and is neither intended to diagnose any
physical or mental condition nor to serve as a substitute for
informed medical advice or care.
Please contact your health professional for medical advice and
treatment. Neither author nor publisher can be held liable by
any person for any loss or damage whatsoever which may arise
from the use of this book or any of the information therein.

Published by
Findhorn Press
117-121 High Street,
Forres IV36 1AB,
Scotland, UK

t +44 (0)1309 690582
f +44 (0)131 777 2711
e info@findhornpress.com
www.findhornpress.com

CONTENTS

Introduction 9

PART ONE – THEORY

1. Why Do Western Women Have Such
   A Bad Time During Menopause? 12
2. The Two Ways to Go Through Menopause
   (and Why Nobody Mentions the Second) 16
3. Western Diets Versus Eastern Health. Is It That Simple? 21
4. The Amazing Ways We Achieve Hormonal Balance 28
5. What We Thought Was Going Wrong
   and How We Have Tried to Fix It 31
6. How We Are Slowly Learning What
   Plant Hormones Can Do For Us 36
7. How We Can Mimic Traditional Diets in Modern Ways.
   Practical Suggestions Backed by Scientific Research 43
8. Why Grow Sprouted Greens and Beans as HRT? In Which, I Put
   All That We Have Learnt So Far Into Historical Perspective 48

PART TWO – EXPERIENCE

9. My Menopause Diary 56
10. Lisa Pope's Menopause Story 68
11. Kate Tym's Menopause Story 70
12. Viryapuspa Nolan's Menopause Story 76
13. Joanne Edward's Menopause Story 81

PART THREE – APPLICATION

14. How Much Do I Need to Take? How Much Am I
    Getting Already? 86
15. All of the Symptoms and More! 88
16. What Can You Do If It Doesn't Work? 104
17. Synthetic Hormones, Chemical Hormones. What Are They?
    Where Are They? And Why You Should Avoid Them 110
18. Hormone-Rich Recipes and Dining Suggestions 118
    Old-Fashioned Recipes 126

PART FOUR – PRACTICAL

19. What Is Sprouting? How Do I Do It? 134
20. How to Grow Mung, Lentil, Aduki, and Chickpea Sprouts 142
21. How to Grow Alfalfa, Broccoli, Radish,
    and Red Clover Sprouts 145
22. How to Grow Fenugreek and Flaxseed (Linseed) Sprouts 149
23. How to Grow Cress 153
24. FAQs and Troubleshooting 156

PART FIVE – DIGGING DEEPER

1. The History of Conventional HRT 163
2. Supplements: Why the Evidence Is So Contradictory
   (and What to Do If You Need to Take Them) 167
3. Bioidentical Hormones (Also Called Bio-Matching or BHRT) 170
4. The Hard Evidence About Endocrine-Disrupting
   Chemicals in the Environment 172
5. Why Haven't Chemical and Industrial
   Hormone Mimics Been Banned? 175
6. List of Estrogenic Foods 178
7. List of Progesteronic Foods 182

   Resources and Interesting Sites 186
   Bibliography 187
   List of Photos 189
   Acknowledgements 190
   About the Author 193
   End Notes 194

DEDICATION

To my mother, **Greta Joyce Watts** –
I wish we had known all this when you were alive.

Introduction

In laboratories all around the world, scientists are peering down their microscopes at little green plants and shoots that are just a few days to a week old. This is because, even though these sprouted seeds and beans have been grown without soil, they are at their peak of nutrition. But most importantly, they contain PLANT HORMONES.

Companies pay scientists to measure their contents, test their growing conditions, isolate their active ingredients, and assess their health effects, so that they can be put into supplements and drugs and sold to us as an alternative to Hormone Replacement Therapy (HRT).

They then write papers on the marvellous benefits of sprouted foods and show how brilliant they are against menopause symptoms, cancer, osteoporosis, heart problems, and dementia.

I wonder, do any of the researchers look at those little sprouts and greens and think about eating them themselves? Do they sneak a few out of the lab and pop them in their sandwiches? Do they start growing them at home? Do they tell their friends to?

I don't know the answer to that. What I do know is that we evolved eating plant hormones, and lots of illnesses have only become common since we stopped. Instead of buying supplements and taking drugs, *we* can all grow them again ourselves. *We* can all harvest the benefits. *We* can grow all our own HRT.

Who Am I?

My name is Sally, and I'm an ex stand-up comic turned health food teacher, and when I started researching the role of plant hormones in menopause I was amazed by what I found out—and you will be, too! In this book, I will show you the science behind what stops our ovaries from working properly, and what to do to help. I will show how healthy postmenopausal women don't need to take artificial hormones; that we can create our own special form of estrogen, which is good for our hair, skin, and vaginas. I will even show why some postmenopausal women finally start having multiple orgasms and others dry up and wither away!

As I was researching, questions kept bugging me. Over and over again, I asked myself, why has it come down to someone like me to tell the world that we can grow our own HRT?

Then I realized that no-one has got a financial interest in getting women to grow their own plant hormones—not the HRT industry, not the supplement makers, not the soya marketers.

This is why it's taken an outsider, an ex stand-up comic with no vested interest beyond wanting to find a solution to my own health problems, to look at things in a new way. This book references over 400 different scientific studies. Everything I am saying here has been proven by science, sometimes many times over. I had to do it this way. I am not a scientist, so I have to be doubly sure of what I am saying.

The truth is, instead of buying supplements and taking drugs, we can all grow all our own HRT. I will show you how simple it is. You don't need a garden or any soil; just a small space, such as a kitchen counter or windowsill. We can all harvest the benefits. We can eat the kind of foods that we evolved on. It's cheaper, healthier, and more natural. In short, it's the way we were meant to be.

PART ONE
– THEORY –

CHAPTER 1

WHY DO WESTERN WOMEN HAVE SUCH A BAD TIME DURING MENOPAUSE?

Why do some societies see menopause symptoms as a disease of modernity? Why do researchers find that in some traditional societies, women don't have a word for menopause and look baffled when asked about hot flushes? Why was the word "menopause" only invented in 1821? Why do Japanese women only get menopause symptoms when they adopt a Western lifestyle? Why do some doctors refer to menopause as a disease, when it happens to half the population?

These were all questions I set out to answer, when I hit 50 and had my first hot flush. I already knew there were such things as Hormone Replacement Therapy (HRT), but I didn't fancy taking pills made from pregnant horse's urine. I heard I could make myself some menopause cake and eat it every day for the next 10 years, and also that there were supplements I could buy from the chemist containing plant hormones that were very expensive.

But what was really bothering me was why do we need to do all this? None of these things were available a hundred years ago. What did females do for the millions of years that we have been evolving? What went wrong with evolution that gives us such a dreadful time?

"Well, of course, it's because we never used to live this long," says one (male!) scientist friend of mine. "Women were old at 30 and dead at 40."

I was intrigued. Were we really only meant to live as long as we could reproduce? Is that it? Are older women no longer viable?

I checked it out, and it's simply not true. One study found that all those horrible "the average age of death was 36" statistics are because infant mortality and women dying during childbirth was so high that it brings down the overall average. Whereas studies into the modal age of adult death, which looks at when you are most likely to die, found that if a hunter-gatherer could survive childhood and giving birth, then they had a big chance of making it to 70.[1]

If there's any doubt, we just need to look to the fossil record. Researchers found that even Neanderthals lived long enough to experience menopause.[2]

Archaeologists can also tell that it was at least 30,000 years ago that human beings started living longer, which coincided with an explosion of both population and cultural innovations such as art and pottery.[3] This gave rise to the "Grandmother" theory—the idea that having older women around is both advantageous for the survival of their grandchildren and to pass on complex skills, such as art and culture.

This, of course, is lovely for our offspring and our artistic natures, but does that mean that women have had at least 30,000 years of hot flushes?

I talk to my scientist friend again.

"Yeah, probably," he says, "because humans are the only primates to menopause. No other animals do. We haven't evolved enough to cope with it!"

This worried me. Are we freaks of nature? Did evolution overstep the mark? Are older women paying the price with hot flushes, osteoporosis, heart disease, and cancer?

So I checked it out and found that he was wrong again! Although we used to believe that humans were the only ones to go through menopause, a recent study at an American primate centre pointed out that apes and monkeys do, too; it's just less obvious because they don't have a regular pattern of menstrual bleeding. That doesn't mean that menopause doesn't happen.[4]

Since then, other researchers have found that it's not just primates, either; whales, dolphins, and even rats go through menopause. And here's the interesting thing—some of them help out with the grandchildren. One study found that "bottlenose dolphins and pilot whales babysit, guard, and even breastfeed their grandchildren."[5] Yes, breast feed! As an older woman I find that very impressive indeed. Not all species are so helpful. Rats, who as I said, also stop being fertile,[6] don't bother to help out at all. But that's rats for you.

It all means that evolution did not make a mistake. Females everywhere can be useful post-reproductively, and interestingly, can get by without any pills, patches, hormonal creams, or injections. You don't see old monkeys unable to swing through the trees because they've got osteoporosis or are having a hot flush. So why can't modern women in Western societies get by?

Are we spoilt? Are we looking for problems? Or are we having a complete-ly different experience to women in traditional societies and our monkey cousins?

Most books and websites say that menopause happens when the number of eggs we have is so low that the ovaries can't respond when our brain hormones, (what's known as the hypothalamus, pituitary axis or HPA) tell them it's time to hatch.

Jenni Murray, in her book *Is It Me or Is It Hot in Here?*, says: "As the supply of eggs in the ovaries dwindles ... the pituitary gland recognizes what's happening and frantically increases its production of FSH, in an attempt to kick-start the reproductive system as normal. As things progress, other symptoms such as flushes and sweats begin." [7]

Gynaecologist John Lee, MD, in his book, *What Your Doctor May Not Tell You About Menopause*, is even more dramatic. "The hypothalamus be-gins 'shouting,' trying to tell the pituitary to tell the ovaries to ovulate." [8]

It's not just hot flushes and night sweats, either, he says. We will also get "mood swings, fatigue, feelings of being cold, and inappropriate responses to other stressors."

And that's just going through menopause. When our periods stop alto-gether, the descriptions get even worse. We have dry skin, sagging libidos, and are more prone to osteoporosis, cancer, heart problems, and dementia.

In the 1960s, gynaecologist Robert Wilson argued that menopause was "living decay" and stated that all postmenopausal women were "diseased castrates." He pronounced that menopause was a result of ovarian failure, which led to, what he called, estrogen deficiency disease. This, he argued, was what was causing all the menopausal symptoms, not just those men-tioned above but suicidal thoughts, depression and frigidity, too. Although, let's be honest. If a doctor told you that you were going to become a dis-eased castrate, you'd get depressed, too.

None of this sounds like a good prospect, and the way Robert Wilson writes you really think this happens to all women, everywhere.

Except it doesn't.

There are lots of women who don't get menopause symptoms. Famously, Japanese and Chinese women don't even have a word for menopause. There are studies of women in traditional societies all over the world showing them alive, well, strong, healthy, and blissfully unaware of what hot flushes are. One commentator, writing in 1897,[9] observed Native American and

Eskimo women failed to find any noteworthy experience of menopause.[10] Later studies in Mayan women found that the only sign of menopause is the end of menstruation.[11]

So my next questions is: Why can't we all do this? What is happening in the bodies of women who menopause without symptoms that makes them do so well? I couldn't find the answer in any of the standard textbooks or internet sites that talk about menopause. So I started searching the hard-core science websites, where research centres publish their findings. There, I found another scenario for the way women menopause. The shocking thing is not just that it exists but that no-one outside the science world has heard about it.

CHAPTER 2

The Two Ways to Go Through Menopause (and Why Nobody Mentions the Second)

In 1966, when Robert Wilson published his book *Feminine Forever*, he stated that all menopausal women needed to take HRT. As we have seen, he argued that postmenopausal women were "castrates" and that menopause was "nature's defeminization." The book was sponsored by the pharmaceutical company producing HRT and, scientific papers published at the time seemed to back up his theory.[12,13]

Even so, not everyone believed him. There was, and still is, a massive backlash.

Just the name of the book upset some women, before they'd even read all the hideous descriptions he gives of our breasts and genitals shrivelling if we don't take HRT. As Jenni Murray points out, though, he only talks about female decline and never mentions "balding, paunchy, creaking middle-aged men and their own living decay."

Also women began asking the same question I have been asking. If menopause symptoms are a disease, why didn't it happen to our grandmothers and great-grand mothers? The feminist movement took this on and argued that they must have just toughed it out and if we do get a few menopause symptoms we should do the same. Women on HRT were accused of artificially trying to turn the clock back. Menopause went from something housewives whispered about to being a hot political issue.

Before we jump on Robert Wilson's grave (he is deceased now), let's look at how he reached his conclusions. He had women sitting in his office saying they couldn't sleep for burning up, they were irritable, they had thinning skin and sagging libidos. In the longer term, he was seeing older women with osteoporosis, heart problems, cancer, and dementia. Women were asking him what to do. So he tested their hormones, saw that they

16

were low on estrogen, told them they had ovarian failure, and tried to fix it. You can actually see that he was really trying to help.

The problem was, however, that Robert Wilson just focussed on the women who came to him because they were feeling ill. When he announced that menopause was a disease, he was assuming all women had ovarian failure and couldn't create the necessary hormones for well-being. He hadn't noticed the healthy, happy women strolling by his window who didn't need to book an appointment with him. Neither had he looked abroad or studied the women in traditional societies having a grand old age without his assistance.

If he had, he might have started questioning why, if all postmenopausal women are suffering from ovarian failure and an inability to make estrogen, then where were these healthy women getting their hormones from? Also, if menopausal symptoms are triggered by the ovaries packing up and the hypothalamus-pituitary-adrenal axis (the HPA axis in the brain responsible for manufacturing the hormones) screaming at them to get going again, why aren't these women getting side effects when their ovaries stop working?

The first clue that something different might be happening is in Dr. John Lee's book, *What Your Doctor May Not Tell You About Menopause*. The book is 500 pages long, and there is just one sentence that points to an alternative. He says that the HPA axis in "some women" stops producing hormones *before* the ovaries wind down. This is hugely important, because if the HPA axis (or hormones produced by the brain) wind down before the ovaries do, then they have no need to scream at the ovaries to keep working, with all the side effects that causes. John Lee, MD, actually states that his own clinical experience showed that, in this scenario, he saw "fewer menopause symptoms."

Of course! The hormones being produced in these women's brains are winding down gently, along with the ovaries, rather than goading them to keep working and getting all the side effects. John Lee mentioned a hormone called GnRH being involved in this process. I quickly found out that it means gonadotropin-releasing hormone. We've been talking about the HPA axis telling the ovaries to produce hormones, but this was a step back from that. GnRH actually tells the brain to tell the ovaries to produce the hormones. In other words, I'd found the über controller!

This gave me something new to search on. So I typed GnRH into Google, along with the word "menopause," and there it all was, ready for me. I'd been researching for over a year at this stage, and because I was now used to reading scientific papers, I'd even say it is easy to see there was another, much gentler scenario for menopause.

The alternative model is where the ovaries keep working for as long as our brain hormones or specifically the GnRH tells them to. The HPA axis doesn't have to "scream" at the poor old ovaries to try and get them going; *it actually tells them when it's time to go through menopause,* tells them they can relax and stop ovulating. The hormones and ovaries all transition slowly together, a much more natural, graceful aging process, with no hot flushes, no moodiness, no horrible dryness. The only mystery is, why has this never got into the public domain?

It turns out that a number of studies have challenged the belief that ovarian failure is the only way to menopause.[14,15,16,17] In 2010, a symposium on reproductive aging (yes, there was a whole symposium on it!) concluded that there is a convincing body of literature supporting the role of the HPA axis, independent of the ovaries during menopause.[18]

None of this research, however, was sponsored by the menopause industry. It was the fertility industry and researchers into aging generally who were giving their attention to this subject. It was those two groups who sponsored the 2010 symposium.

In fact, as far back as 1964 (two years before Robert Wilson produced his book), scientists were proving that the ovaries did not always take the lead role in menopause.[19]

One study is particularly interesting because they took old, supposedly defunct ovaries and implanted them in younger animals, and they started working again, proving that it's the hormones produced by the brain that are most important in menopause. In 1972 a team tried the opposite and gave the HPA axis hormones from old rats to young rats with functioning ovaries, and they stopped working.[20] From these studies it seems obvious that a true menopause is directed by the brain, the HPA axis driven by GnRH.

Menopause symptoms only happen when the ovaries fail before the hormones produced in the brain have decided it's time to stop. Our HPA axis doesn't understand why the ovaries aren't responding and keeps nagging them, upping their hormone levels, with unpleasant side effects.

This shouldn't be the rule; this should be the exception, and as we have seen in some countries it is. The only true menopause symptom is erratic periods, as hormones slowly rebalance themselves. Interestingly enough, even rats get this symptom.[21]

So given the right circumstances, it seems that ovaries can go on for as long as we need them.[22] This is important, because even after we menopause we do need them. A healthy postmenopausal ovary still creates lots of hormones for us. The ultimate proof that we still need our ovaries comes from all the women who had their ovaries removed, which sadly, used to be done routinely, when postmenopausal women had hysterectomies. Doctors assumed that because we didn't menstruate we didn't need them.

However, a number of studies[23, 24] concluded that this is very wrong. One study found that removal of the ovaries is "associated with higher risks of coronary artery disease, stroke, hip fracture, Parkinson's, dementia, cognitive impairment, depression, and anxiety."[25] This is particularly noteworthy because women can easily be supplemented with artificial estrogen, but it seems nothing works as well as our own ovaries, which even for older women are still central to our hormonal wellbeing.

The interesting thing is that the list of side effects experienced by women who have had their ovaries removed is very similar to those symptoms described by Robert Wilson. There is no doubt that some women do suffer from unnatural ovarian failure and cannot make the hormones they need, and these were the women who ended up in his clinics. It seems that if our ovaries fail totally, and we don't get the right hormones, we might indeed suffer terribly. This is not the norm, though. Many women's ovaries keep working and producing what the brain hormones made through the HPA demands of them.

It's a shame that Robert Wilson never questioned why his patients' ovaries were not working. He never tried, at least in the first instance, to get them going again, and instead, chose to give them HRT. Perhaps because many of his clients seemed to respond well to the estrogen replacement therapy, he pronounced it a wonder cure and thought he had the elixir of life. It took a while to establish the link between estrogen therapy and cancer, but by then it was too late. His book had sold 10 million copies, menopause was seen by doctors as a disease, and HRT was touted as the cure.

Meanwhile, the backlash led by the feminist movement went to the other extreme. They pronounced menopause symptoms to be a natural phenomenon that good feminist women should just ignore. Germaine Greer, in her book *The Change*, said that many women don't go to the doctor for their menopause symptoms because of "their attitude to doctors, and their coping style rather than to the extent to which they experience symptoms." [26] She further stated that the "bewildering array of symptoms" were produced by women who had "internalized their rage." I think it must have been really hard for women with terrible symptoms to read statements like that.

What neither side realized was that they were both right. There were some women who, as Robert Wilson suggested, have ovarian failure and terrible symptoms, and some women who have a natural menopause, during which their ovaries keep working until the end with no symptoms. And there are probably many stages in between. Now that we know this, we can perhaps be more generous to those whose ovaries have failed and have had to turn to HRT, and feel grateful if we have not. How bad our menopausal symptoms are will depend on how much function our ovaries still have.

There is yet to be a specific study comparing the two models of menopause: the gentle wind-down versus the premature ovarian failure. I guess when this becomes more generally known, instead of rushing to get HRT, women will start asking how they can get their ovaries working again. Younger women will want to know how they can keep their ovaries going for as long as possible. And we will all be asking what causes ovaries to fail in the first place.

According to Dr. John Lee, the final wind-down of hormones is a "genetically programmed change" akin to how the body knows when to begin menstruation. This is the natural way. It's what we used to do in the past. It's what women in traditional societies do seamlessly. So the big question is, why can't we all do it now?

CHAPTER 3

Western Diets Versus Eastern Health. Is It That Simple?

For years, both scientists and anthropologists have been pondering the different experiences of menopause around the world, and a number of studies have been undertaken. Of these, what has become known as the "Japanese study" [27] is undoubtedly the most famous. It was carried out by intrepid researcher Margaret Lock, who produced several papers on why Japanese women lacked a special word for menopause, or more importantly, the symptoms to go with it.

Then she asked the question everyone wanted to know. Why?

Her further research[28] showed that both traditional Thai and Chinese women were also enjoying trouble-free menopause. She speculated that the Asian diet of "vegetables, seaweed, fish, and soya" was giving them a rich mix of vitamins, minerals, trace elements, and something not many people had heard of at the time: plant estrogen. She noted the long tradition of herbalism in these countries, and that the women she studied all took regular weight-bearing exercise. She also cited the fact that many of the women live in multi-generation households where the elderly are highly respected, and wondered whether this was a factor for aging gracefully.

However there were no headlines saying, "Respect your elders to banish hot flushes?" Or "eat fish, veg, and seaweed for fewer menopause symptoms". Or even "Herbalism works!"

What excited everyone, particularly the marketing men, was soya, and they set to work persuading us that Japanese women had this amazing special food, which contained plant estrogens. They introduced us to the word "isoflavones," which is the estrogenic part of the bean, and told us that it was saving Japanese women from the ravages of menopausal symptoms and diseases of old age.

Some learned commentators did point out that the Japanese miracle might not just be about the soya, but nobody listened. It soon became the "Eastern Wonder Food." Health-conscious women started looking for ways to eat more of it. The food industry responded by making soya sausages, burgers, milk, and yoghurt, while at the same time soya was being added to flour and many general products such as bread, cakes, and cereals. Whether we wanted it or not, we were all suddenly eating soya.

Strangely, the reverse was happening in the cities of Japan itself, where it was becoming fashionable to swap to a Westernized diet. However, it wasn't long before the women concerned started getting Western-style menopause symptoms to go along with it.[29,30] When this first happened, Japanese women were accused of being spoilt, and menopause symptoms were seen as a "disease of luxury." It took a while for everyone to realize that it was about the change in diet.

Meanwhile, in the West, the soya revolution was in full swing. One article promoting soya opened with the words, "Just imagine you could grow the perfect food. This food not only would provide affordable nutrition but also would be delicious and easy to prepare in a variety of ways. It would be a healthful food, with no saturated fat."[31]

Who could resist that? And if you found that you couldn't bear to eat soya, you could buy supplements that contained the active ingredient (isoflavones) instead.

The marketing ploy for the pills was to point to research showing that women with more plant estrogen in their *diets* have fewer menopause symptoms; it didn't mention that this might not be the case for *supplements*. However, studies into supplements were immediately commissioned, and a few did manage to show improvement. Strangely, these were often the ones sponsored by the supplement manufacturers. Rarely could the independent studies produce the same results;[32] at their best being very random, and at their worst, showing no improvement whatsoever.[33]

By 2003, there had been so many studies carried out you could almost say anything you liked about isoflavones and plant estrogens and find research to back it up. To combat this, there have been a number of meta analyses of studies done over time.

Appendix 2 looks at all the research in detail, but the overall conclusion was unequivocal: women who consume plant hormones as part of their diets don't get menopause symptoms specifically, and are in very good health generally. Supplements on the other hand "are much less effective than dietary sources." [34] None of this made any difference. Sales of both soya and supplements rocketed but consumers still weren't being told the whole story.

Firstly, soya is not the only food that contains plant estrogens in the form of isoflavones. In the 1920s, when researchers discovered a way to measure it, they found isoflavones in so many foods (over 300 in fact) that they thought their machine was broken. If you eat any kind of bean and most vegetables, you will be taking in isoflavones. In fact, supplement makers didn't only use soya to extract plant estrogen; they also used other highly estrogenic plants, such as red clover and alfalfa, which at least had the advantage that it alerted people like me that there was another way to get it.

Secondly, isoflavones are not the only plant hormones around. Compounds called lignans and coumestrol are also highly estrogenic. Lignans are generally found in green vegetables, but particularly in seaweed, which is the second highest source of it in the world,[35] and we all know how much the Japanese like to eat seaweed. Coumestrol, which, by the way, is 35–50 percent stronger than isoflavones,[36] is found in alfalfa sprouts, mung bean sprouts, and pea shoots (peas are so rich is coumestrol they used to be known as vitamin P!).

These again are all a big part of the Japanese diet, plus red clover (which is used in Asian herbal medicine) has all three kinds of plant estrogen. It seems the lucky old Japanese were doing everything right. So to give soya and isoflavones all the credit for the many healthy benefits of Japanese cuisine is really quite fraudulent.

Thirdly, whilst soya contains a multitude of vitamins, minerals, and nutrients, it also contains phytic acid, which stops you absorbing them. The effect of phytic acid is so bad that scientists refer to it as an "anti-nutrient."[37] This is why, historically, soya beans were considered to be inedible. They only became fit for human consumption during the Chung Dynasty in 1000 BC, when Asian countries learnt to sprout and ferment them. Sprouting and fermenting soya beans drastically reduces the levels of phytic acid, and in the case of sprouting, increases the vitamin and mineral content as well.

The final blow is that even though the traditional Asian diet uses fermented soya, it is mainly as a side dish; the Japanese eat nowhere near the amounts of soya earnest vegetarians in the West might end up consuming.

This is bad news for those of us who have been diligently eating our soya burgers and drinking our soya milk for years, and I include myself in that category.

Nowadays, in their research, scientists sometimes differentiate between the two ways of eating soya. One study into thyroid cancer found no benefit from consumption of "Western" processed soya foods, which are unfermented, processed, and full of additives. However, they found that "the consumption of traditional and nontraditional soy-based foods and alfalfa sprouts was associated with a reduced risk of thyroid cancer." [38]

Another study suggested that eating tofu (unfermented soya) was linked to an increase in cognitive decline in the elderly, whereas eating tempeh (fermented soya) was linked to enhanced cognitive function in the same age group. [39,40]

Finally, what the promoters of soya have never answered is this: if women need to eat soya to have a healthy menopause, why have menopause symptoms only become commonplace in the West since the industrial revolution? It's not like we used to eat soya and need to bring it back. We never ate it; yet there was no epidemic of menopause symptoms until the twentieth century. It begs the question what did we used to do that stopped us from getting menopause symptoms that we no longer do?

To answer this, we need to research our own traditional diet here in the United Kingdom and the things we no longer eat.

Take, for example, sprouted mustard and cress, hugely popular in Britain since Anglo Saxon times. Even the Victorians loved sprinkling it on their food, and thought of it as their "ginseng."

Traditionally, the mix was 75 percent cress and 25 percent mustard, and both of these sprouts contain lignans for plant estrogen as well as being rich in plant progesterone [41,42] and cancer fighting compounds. [121] However, in the twentieth century, commercial growers replaced this mix with 85 percent rapeseed and 15 percent cress and called it "cress salad" (unfortunately, it's not illegal to do that).

Rapeseed greens always used to be considered inedible due to the high amounts of erucic acid. Modern rape is genetically engineered to have less of this toxic chemical so that it can at least be made into oil but they don't have the rich bounty of cancer-fighting compounds that mustard and cress have. [43]

The producers of genetically modified rapeseed sprouts wouldn't have been thinking about that though. They were probably just trying to cut costs and thought that one green sprout is very like another. Thus, this bland offering can still be found in supermarkets, but people no longer crave it the way they used to love the real thing; perhaps our bodies sense it's not as good. As a result mustard and cress are no longer a normal part of our diets.

Cress is not the only place that we used to get plant hormones from. A French study specifically looked at how Western women get plant estrogen from lignans. These are found in whole grains, beans, berries, nuts and seeds, and especially flaxseed (also known as linseed), which is the richest source of lignans on the planet. This study is important because researchers looked at nearly 60,000 Western women who do not consume soya and concluded that women who ate a lot of lignans had reduced risks of all kinds of postmenopausal breast cancer.[44]

So, while Asian cultures were sprinkling plant hormones on their food in the form of alfalfa sprouts, we in Britain were getting the same from mustard and cress. Whilst the Japanese ate mung beans and soya, we ate peas and beans, full of isoflavones and coumestrol. They ate sesame seeds (also rich in lignans), whilst we ate flaxseeds (linseeds). They ate a wide variety of green vegetables, full of plant hormones and plant nutrients, and so did we. Both Asian herbal medicine[45] and Western folk medicine use red clover as herbal medicine, specifically for menopause symptoms, and again, packed with plant hormones.

Suddenly, the Japanese were still doing all that, but we had started processing our foods and had stopped eating a wide range of vegetables, nuts, beans, and seeds. It looks like that has contributed to our health problems generally and to our menopause symptoms specifically.

If we in Britain had stuck to traditional foods and the Japanese had "modernized" and started living off processed foods, pizza, pasta, and curry and forgotten their heritage, it would have been them with the menopause symptoms and diseases of aging, studying us to see what we were doing right.

Evidence from around the world makes it easy to pinpoint what went wrong. Dr. Andrew F. Currier, writing in 1897, noted that peasants in Scandinavia, Germany, and Russia were "apt to complain little of experiences of the menopause… [while] the highly organized city-bred woman of fashion, women who fret and worry, are apt to experience the disagreeable and annoying features of menopause."[46]

Of course, looking back, we can see that it is richer city women who have abandoned their traditional diet, no doubt thinking that refined foods such as sugar and processed meats were a modern luxury. Meanwhile, the peasants, who would have still been on a traditional diet of legumes and greens and flaxmeal, were sailing through menopause. Even recently, a study of Chinese women found that those in the cities were starting to suffer from menopause symptoms whilst those on the farms were not.[47] Similarly vegetarians living in the West who eat a diet rich in beans, legumes, and vegetables also had less menopause symptoms and interestingly less cancer too.[48]

If you put all this together, successful traditional cultures contained everything they needed for a healthy diet and healthy ovaries. This is because their cultures have evolved over thousands of years, through trial and error and harsh conditions; they know how to produce healthy women, and indeed grandmothers. From that perspective it's no accident that menopause symptoms and these horrible diseases happened when we started moving to towns, and the number of foods we ate became restricted, more processed, and less nutritious as mass farming came into use.

Luckily, we still had some cultures to show us what was normal and what wasn't, and menopause symptoms are not normal. It is not a coincidence that the Industrial Revolution took place between 1789 and 1848,[49] and the word "menopause" was invented in 1821, slap, bang in the middle of it. Before then we talked of a climeratic, which means "time of transition to old age." It equally applied to men and women and ranged between the ages of 45 and 60.

For those of you still wondering whether Margaret Lock's idea that different cultural attitudes to aging, such as respecting the elderly and living in multigenerational households might make a difference, I have this for you.

An American woman called Yewoubdari Beyenene (who I like to think was worrying whether she ought to be living with her own mother) did a study that takes this head on.[50] She looked at two similar peasant cultures, Mayans and Greek. In both of them the elderly have very high status and apparently even look forward to menopause, yet the Greek peasant women have hot flushes and Mayans do not. Beyenene concludes that it is diet and fertility patterns that make the difference and goes on to wonder if there is another model for menopause because "hot flushes are not universal."

Everything I have researched seems to point to a diet rich in plant hormones and nutrients as the key to healthy menopause and old age. We don't have to eat soya to achieve this; we have our own way of doing things, and can combine this with modern sprouting techniques to make up any slack. Interestingly, many Japanese women are reverting to their traditional diet,[51] no matter how rich or sophisticated they are, because otherwise, they fear they will get what they call "Western diseases."

If we go back to my original contention that healthy functioning ovaries are the key to avoiding menopausal symptoms, then it is clearly something to do with modern lifestyle generally and plant hormones specifically that is making the difference. It seems that a traditional diet can really help, but how? To find this out, we first need to understand how we achieve hormonal balance, what can go wrong, and how plant hormones fit into this.

CHAPTER 4

The Amazing Ways We Achieve Hormonal Balance

Lots of commentators have waxed lyrical about the wonders of the female hormonal system. When it works well, it's a dance, a symphony, a harmony, a twirling and a balancing, our hormones, rising and falling, dipping and swelling. But when it goes wrong … oh boy, are we in trouble!

For the first half of our cycle, estrogen builds up womb and breast tissue ready for conception, whilst at the same time the ovaries are busy ripening eggs in their follicles. At the point of ovulation, an egg is dispatched towards the waiting womb. And here's the fascinating bit: the exact site of the empty egg follicle is where we start to manufacture the hormone progesterone.

This progesterone immediately takes over. It clears any excess estrogen from our systems whilst continuing to build up the womb ready for a baby. If there is no fertilization, with no baby to look after, our progesterone levels drop dramatically. This tells the womb to shed its lining, which brings on a period.

The most obvious thing that can go wrong is if we don't ovulate. No ovulation means no empty egg follicle to produce progesterone. Without progesterone, there is nothing to clear out estrogen from our systems, or tell our womb lining when to shed, so it just keeps building up. This can mean long cycles and heavy periods.

If we consistently fail to ovulate, we will become what is known as "estrogen dominant." This term was coined by John Lee, MD, in his book *What Your Doctor May Not Tell You About Menopause*. It basically means you have too much estrogen sloshing around in your system without the progesterone to match it. It can lead to cell growth in our reproductive areas and a whole host of menstrual problems such as endometriosis (build up of womb tissue), fibroids (lumpy tissue attached to the womb), fibrocystic breasts (lumpy tissue attached to the breasts), and of course, infertility. In the long term, scientists have found that lack of ovulation is also associated with osteoporosis, heart disease,[52] and several cancers, such as breast, endometrial, and thyroid.[53, 54, 55]

So ovulating is really important. Even if we don't want to get pregnant, we should welcome ovulation right up to the moment we menopause. We need to keep creating progesterone to keep us healthy. Before I started researching this book, I was looking forward to my periods stopping, but I ended up blessing every one.

Eventually, of course, ovulation does stop, and we will go into full menopause. We have seen that there are two ways to do this. One way is that the hormones made in the brain via the HPA axis gently start telling the ovaries to create less and less hormones until we no longer menstruate. The other is when our ovaries fail and cannot respond to what the brain hormones ask them to do. In the latter case, the body gives us hot flushes, as the brain sends more and more hormonal messages, and as mentioned, is effectively "screaming" at the ovaries to get on with it. The same hormones that control our ovaries control the blood vessels that cause us to be hot or cold. So when we get hot flushes, we literally feel that things are going wrong and, strangely, this might even be a good thing, because otherwise, we wouldn't get a chance to put it right.

Throughout this book, I have been talking about estrogen as if it is just one hormone, but in fact there are lots of different kinds. The three main ones are called estriol, estradiol, and estrione. I think that when scientists were naming them they went for the Huey, Dewey, and Louie effect. But whereas Huey, Dewey, and Louie were triplets of the same age and size, the three estrogens have different strengths and different affinities for different parts of the body.[56]

Estradiol, produced by women in their fertile years, is the strongest estrogen. Estrone is in the middle, coming in at a third to two thirds as strong, whereas estriol, is the weakest, at only an eighth as strong.

Estriol is a very interesting hormone because it the predominant estrogen in older women. Not only is it very gentle and less likely to cause cancer but it has a special affinity with keeping our vaginas, skin, and hair healthy.[57,58] This is fabulous, and it's clear that without it older women might get horrible symptoms such as dryness, sagging libido, and thinning skin. This is why people think of estriol as the special older lady estrogen, but in fact it is also made in massive amounts by pregnant women. Most scientists think that this is to protect the growing foetus from the effects of stronger estrogens, and with its lovely effect on hair and skin, it might also explain why pregnant women start "blooming."

The good news is that the body has a natural ability to convert all the different estrogens to each other. More specifically estrione (the middle one) can be converted to estradiol, whereas estriol (the weakest one) is made from the other two by the liver (which is why liver problems can lead to hormone imbalance). Yet estriol (the weak one) at high doses can act like the other two.[59] This is a marvellous tool for hormonal balance.

And here's the other thing: *we still don't know everything.* For that reason alone, I believe that when we have problems the first thing we should do is to encourage our bodies to rebalance themselves naturally, and as we'll see, that's where plant hormones come in. It's surely folly to think that we can artificially fix such a finely balanced and delicate system, which has evolved over millions of years. However that has never stopped us trying.

CHAPTER 5

WHAT WE THOUGHT WAS GOING WRONG AND HOW WE HAVE TRIED TO FIX IT

So what is going wrong? What is it about the Western world, the Western diet, and the Western lifestyle that so upsets our hormonal balance that a 2015 Norwegian research project reported that a third of women were not ovulating.[52]

The study highlighted several possible reasons, beginning with stress and bad diet. I can hear some of you thinking, *Yeah, yeah. Everything is blamed on stress and bad diet.* So here are the specifics.

Stress depletes the adrenal glands, which after menopause are one of the few ways the body can create its own progesterone. Stress also means we don't digest our food properly, which is important because it hampers the body's ability to convert one hormone to another. To do that we need enzymes, which in turn require vitamins and minerals to work, most notably magnesium, calcium, B vitamins, and vitamin E.[60] So without the right food or the ability to digest it, we can't balance our hormones.[29]

John Lee, MD describes the vicious circle we can get into as this: "Blood sugar becomes constantly unstable. Digestion goes awry, so she isn't absorbing nutrients properly. The ovaries respond by shutting down in favour of survival… progesterone production occurs only at the adrenals but they aren't working."[61] Of course, all this leads to estrogen dominance, with all the potential problems we saw in the last chapter.

The next problem is that we ingest so many artificial estrogens in our water from women on the pill and HRT who are peeing them out.[62] In America, growth hormones are still found in meat and milk, although they are banned in Europe (more about this later).

Plus there are industrially manufactured hormones in pesticides, fungicides, detergents, and plastic, and these all disrupt our hormones. They are known as xenestrogens or EDCs (Endocrine Disrupting Chemicals). Interestingly enough, the pesticide DDT was one of the first to come into mass use in 1939. This was 20 years before Robert Wilson declared that all menopausal women were castrates. Can it be a coincidence, or is this the first generation to be affected by pesticides?

Certainly, American research biologist Rachel Carson thought so. In the 1960s, she wrote her famous book, *Silent Spring,* showing that DDT was feminizing fish and making the shells of eagles' eggs thinner.[63] The chemical industry accused her of being "hysterical" (well, she was a woman) and "unscientific" (even though she was a trained biologist and used scientific studies to support her case). Obviously, it was easy to attack a lone women who dared write a science book (you can see why I'm interested in this). However, she was proved right, and in response, the US government created the Environmental Protection Agency (EPA) in 1970. DDT was the first chemical they banned, in 1972.

You might think the story should end there, but this battle is still going on today, not only over DDT, which is still used in some countries, but over a whole host of different chemicals, pesticides, pollutants, and plastics. The difference now is that the argument is between scientists working for the World Health Organisation (WHO) and those employed by the industrial and chemical industries.

Study after study has warned about these chemicals. Not for nothing are they called endocrine disruptors. They interfere with hormone action.[64] They scramble our hormonal signals.[65] They stop ovarian eggs from maturing.[66] Yes, they are scrambling our eggs. It's enough to put you off your breakfast!

Luckily for us, though, WHO is on to the chemical industry, along with a number of governments, which have banned many of these chemicals, limited their amounts, or restricted their use. There is also a lot you can do to avoid chemicals. Chapter 17 will show you how, and which sprouted foods help clear them from your body.

So industrial chemicals, stress, and processed foods can all upset our ovaries, but this is the modern age in a nutshell. No wonder hormonal problems have been growing. Yet when the pioneers of HRT produced their papers about older women's ovaries not working, there was no talk of a reason that this might be. They made it seem that it was our lot. Getting old made us estrogen deficient, and that this is the price we pay for living longer. How lucky we were that they had a pill to cure us, it was called hormone replacement therapy, or HRT.

Nothing is ever that simple, though. The first obvious problem was that they gave women estrogen without progesterone which, by the 1970s, caused a massive rise in endometrial cancer.[67] Scientists realized that they needed progesterone in the mix to give a better hormonal balance, and the production of a progesterone pill became big business. Pharmaceutical companies already knew how to make progesterone from a strain of wild Mexican yams that contain a compound called diosgenin, but it was so similar to human progesterone that it couldn't be patented, as you can't patent something that exists naturally.

What happened next is subject to debate. We do know that scientists had already found ways to add extra molecules to the progesterone mix, which meant it could be patented, and it was this kind of synthetic progesterone that was added to HRT. Since then, millions of prescriptions have been filled, and today, if you get traditional HRT from your doctor, you will most likely be given synthetic progesterone to go with it. The more natural form without the extra molecules was sidelined. Hardly anyone used it, except for the fertility industry, which found that the synthetic kind simply didn't work for making babies.

That much is agreed upon. What is controversial is why and how the extra molecules got there. Obviously, it looks like the pharmaceutical industry wanted to make money. Some in the science world have strenuously denied this, and indeed, seem offended that they should be accused of such skulduggery. However, they fail to offer any other explanation as to why you would make something that is natural, less so. In the short term, the synthetic progesterone did seem to help,[68] but long term, it increased the risks of cardiovascular disease, heart attack, stroke, and breast cancer.[69] [70] It seems that every time we interfered to solve one problem, we in turn created a whole load more.[71,72,]

Other problems with HRT took longer to tease out. In the early noughties, three large HRT trials were started. They followed thousands of perimenopausal and postmenopausal women placed on HRT, whether they had symptoms or not. This was a really bad move. Within three years, trials were sensationally cancelled, as they showed women on HRT had increased rates of cancer, heart disease, and thrombosis. However, with hindsight, they have realized that it was mainly giving HRT to women *without* symptoms that was the problem. Clearly, these women were happily creating enough hormones of their own and giving them more on top of that was a disaster.

Strangely, at long last, this is acknowledgement that many women do create enough hormones of their own and do not need HRT. Menopause is not a universal deficiency disease, and indeed, it is dangerous overkill to start giving some women extra hormones.

Today, if you go to your doctor with menopause symptoms, you will likely be offered HRT, but only if you are under 60 and don't smoke, have high blood pressure, or a family history of breast cancer or thrombosis. Otherwise, you might not be given it, even if you beg. If you do go on HRT, you will be advised to come off it before you are 60, because the risk factors rise sharply after that. At this point, your doctor will have no more medicine for you, although they might offer you antidepressants!

So what happens then?

Lots of scientists are now wondering whether plant hormones are the solution. John Lee, MD, the first doctor to recognize "estrogen dominance," thought they were. His book *What Your Doctor May Not Tell You About Menopause,* a best-seller, offered another take on this unlikely hot topic.

As we have seen, Dr. Lee argued that many women are suffering from estrogen dominance and described 33 illnesses that are caused or impacted as a result. Some of them are quite vague illnesses, such as fatigue, depression, weight gain, water retention, headache, mood swings, inability to handle stress, and loss of libido, all of which could equally be caused by a hangover or indeed a bad marriage!

However some are more specific, such as uterine fibroids, endometriosis, low metabolism, hypothyroidism, fibrocystic breasts, unstable blood sugar, and being cold all the time.[73] In this respect, Dr. Lee's view is similar to that of Robert Wilson: there's nothing like giving women a list of horrible illnesses they might get to keep us interested!

The answer proposed by Dr. Lee was (I'm talking past tense, because he is deceased) to use natural progesterone cream made from plants and plant hormones. It was available on his website, and yes, he did have shares in the company. In simple terms, upping your progesterone to match higher estrogen levels looks like an obvious answer, the way traditional HRT did in the early days. His book gives many case studies. There's no hint that a single patient had any problem with progesterone cream, and he wrote that we could all take it until we are 99 years old. If you search the internet, however, there are lots of testimonials from women stating what a terrible time they had using natural progesterone, and a couple of double-blind studies have found the cream ineffective compared with a placebo.[74,75]

I believe there is a place for natural hormones, including progesterone cream. However, the problem with upping our progesterone to match ever rising estrogen levels is that it still doesn't solve the problem of women not ovulating in the first place. When we ovulate, we create our own progesterone and don't need to take the synthetic kind. Older women who have stopped menstruating are never going to produce that much progesterone and are never going to ovulate again; yet, as we have discussed, women in traditional societies have a healthy old age, without paying for progesterone cream until they are 99. So just how are they doing it?

Herbalists have always said that certain plants such as red clover, sage, thyme, black cohosh and wild yam can raise progesterone.[76] All have been used by women for thousands of years in different cultures to combat menstrual problems. Dr. Lee hinted at the answer himself in his book, when he wrote that in non-industrial countries "whose diets are rich in fresh vegetables, all sorts of progesterone deficiency is rare." We are back to diet again and specifically those that contain high amounts of plant hormones.

I know that when women come off HRT, some doctors unofficially (and sometimes even officially) recommend plant hormones. They might casually mention that Asian women have fewer menopause problems, and it might be because they eat a lot of them. If you have been through menopause, been told to take HRT, and have come out the other side only to be told about plant hormones, it does beg the question: Could they have saved you in the first place? Much of the research about plant hormones is relatively new, and I think that doctors simply don't know about it, or else they would tell women about plant hormones *before* they put them on HRT. Let's see why.

CHAPTER 6

How We Are Slowly Learning What Plant Hormones Can Do For Us

"So plants have hormones. Does that mean they get moody if we don't water them?" asks a friend of mine when I tell him I'm writing this book.

No, I tell him, because the big news is that although we call them plant hormones, there aren't any actual hormones in the plants themselves. The different kinds of plant estrogen that I talked about earlier (isoflavones, lignans, and coumestrol) are converted into hormones by our own gut bacteria.

I usually have to explain it again, because it's just so amazing. When we eat certain plants and beans, our bodies create plant estrogen and progesterone from them. Yes, we have our own little pharmacy inside us. All we have to do is feed it the right foods. It is enough to make the pills in your bathroom cabinet very jealous indeed!

There are a number of ways that plant hormones work. Most of the studies are on plant estrogen, so let's go with that first.

We all have estrogen receptors in each of our cells. Some of them are calming receptors, and some of them stimulating. They are actually designed for our own estrogen, but other estrogens can fight each other, to get on them. Plant estrogen is much weaker than that created by our ovaries. If we have too much estrogen in our systems, the plant estrogen will be attracted to the calming receptors and will offer a very low dose of estrogen, as little as a thousandth of the strength of our own. Yet if we don't have enough estrogen, it will be attracted to our stimulating receptors and will offer a stronger dose at least a third as strong.[77]

This is very clever. It means that plant estrogen can be both estrogenic and anti-estrogenic.[78] It really is nature's hormone replacement therapy.

We have already seen that estriol, that special postmenopausal hormone is only an eighth as strong as a fertile woman's estrogen, so plant estrogen

36

exerting an influence a third as strong could be very important for older women who might be deficient. Added to this, plant hormones exert different strengths depending on where the receptors are in the body, so they are stronger in the uterus and weaker in the pituitary.[79] It's amazing that they are actually fine-tuned to what different parts of our bodies need. What a marvellous tool for hormonal balance.

Sadly, plant hormones aren't the only thing attracted to our estrogen receptors. Remember, we talked about industrial xenestrogens and EDCs, endocrine disruptors, in Chapter 5. Well, they too can attach to our estrogen receptors and can do anything from simply blocking other estrogens to more insidiously, sending out the wrong signals to our reproductive systems. If this were a movie script, I would be playing dark music now, because these really are the baddies. Luckily, plant hormones (the goodies, cue swelling orchestral music) fight them to get on our receptors instead. The Greek name for plant estrogens is "phytoestrogens." I like to think of them as fighting estrogens! Fighting off those industrial and chemical estrogens and keeping our bodies healthy.

For a long time we thought what I just described was the only way that plant hormones worked, but in 2015, a study found that we actually have special receptors in our bodies, just looking for plant estrogen.[80] Scientists had known about this receptor's existence for a long time but they didn't know what it was receiving, so they referred to it as an "orphan" receptor. They have a whole orphanage of other receptors waiting to be identified, too, and it's easy to wonder if some of them might be receiving other plant hormones. The search is underway right now in labs around the world, so it's all still to be discovered.[81]

This potentially can give the body another way of controlling hormones, and of always being able to access the weaker plant estrogens when it needs to. It's a fantastic concept, and it shows how important plant hormones are, that our bodies know what to do with them all, *and is actually looking for them.*

The reason we still don't know everything is because even though plant hormones are millions of years old, we only started discovering them in 1926 and then it was just plant estrogen in the form of isoflavones. Lignans were found shortly after, whilst coumestrol was not identified until 1957.

As for plant progesterone, for a long time it was thought not to exist at all. Herbalists have always said that wild yam contains plant progesterone and have encouraged women to use wild yam cream, but proper scientific tests showed it was useless.[82] As a result, those touting it were accused of quackery, and plant progesterone was seen to be a myth.

Luckily, scientific observation never stops! In 2008, a team at the University of Illinois in Chicago were testing the effects of plant estrogen by feeding large amounts to rats that have no ovaries, which meant that the rats could not create any of their own hormones to interfere with the results. (It's an interesting point that if scientists want to give the rats cancer, they feed them too much estrogen; if they want to give them osteoporosis, they give them too little, which in itself shows how important hormonal balance is.) [121]

Anyway, the team were specifically feeding rats large amounts of isoflavones extracted from both red clover and hops. The rats responded as they always do, with the kind of cell proliferation that can lead to cancer. However, when they were fed with an extract made from the WHOLE red clover plant, the rats were protected from this effect. Something in the whole plant was balancing their systems. Could it be that these plants contained progesterone too?

In 2012, another team carried out more studies on eight different herbs and foods that are traditionally used for hormonal balance. They discovered that two compounds—kaempferol, found in red clover, and apigenin, found in chaste tree berry—were having a progesteronic effect.[83] They noted that of the two, kaempferol was the most active. This study was only in the petri dish, which doesn't always mean that things can work in the body. So more tests were commissioned that tested kaempferol from red clover in rats and concluded that it was having a progesteronic effect.[84]

What excited the scientists is that this means that red clover not only contains all the different forms of plant estrogen but has plant progesterone as well. No wonder it has been used for thousands of years to help hormonal balance. And yes, as well as red clover, plant progesterone is in all of the plants herbalists said it was, such as sage and black cohosh.

A fourth study is now underway on plant progesterone (kaempferol and apigenin), covering safety, impact, and its interaction with other plant hormones. [85] This is a very exciting area of research and could change the way we think about plant estrogen and plant progesterone.

Scientists have known about kaempferol for a while. There are a number of studies showing that it has enormous health benefits against all those illnesses that we in the West worry about so much, including cancer, heart disease, diabetes, and osteoporosis.[86] The pharmaceutical industry is keenly investigating how it can harness the power of kaempferol to create anti-cancer drugs. One research project noted that "kaempferol is much less toxic to normal cells in comparison to standard chemotherapy drugs."[87]

Other studies have specifically looked at kaempferol's effect on colon cancer,[88] bladder cancer,[89] and ovarian cancer.[90] However, according to a 2013 overview of all the different kaempferol studies, they are not even near producing a drug yet.[86]

Apigenin is also getting a lot of attention from scientists. It may be weaker in terms of its progesteronic impact, but (in the petri dish) it has been shown to stop cancer cells from spreading and, in fact, tells them to die![91]

Sprouts that contain kaempferol as well as red clover are alfalfa, mustard, cress, and broccoli.[41,92] As they have some plant estrogens, too (even the brassicas have lignans), they really are your complete hormonal package.[93]

Fenugreek not only has kaempferol but it's high in apigenin, and it even has diosgenin, too.[94] As you'll see in Appendix 5, it's very rare to find diosgenin outside of wild yams, and despite those early tests, scientists have now discovered that our bodies can create plant progesterone from it after all. What the early research didn't take into account is the role of gut bacteria in making hormones, which, of course, is the same way we make all the other plant hormones![95]

If this were a novel, it would get even more exciting at this point, because scientists think that red clover may contain something else that is providing progesterone and protecting our systems, but, and here's where the plot thickens, they don't know what! Basically, elderly rats were fed an extract made from the whole red clover plant, and scientists measured the effects. They couldn't understand why such small amounts of kaempferol were having such a big impact, and the study had to conclude that some other factor within the plant must be having a protective effect.[96]

This is the reason we must not isolate plant nutrients, otherwise, as one study notes, "we might miss complementary relationships between compounds in plant extracts".[97] It seems that we need both plant estrogen and plant progesterone. One study concluded that the use of one without the other might increase the risk of developing endometrial hyperplasia and cancer in the same way as conventional HRT did when it consisted of estrogen alone.[83]

This is an important point. If you read the University of Seville's overview of kaempferol, you'll see the lists of the amazing health benefits I have mentioned above, [41] but here's the big thing: the foods that contain kaempferol are also packed with many other vitamins, minerals, and phytochemicals (including plant estrogen) that might be helping out as well. This is because kaempferol is found in fruits and vegetables in general, and raw greens in particular, so when you eat them, you get a wealth of other plant chemicals that will all be working away, doing their bit, to help you.

What makes plant chemicals (or phytochemicals as scientist call them) so exciting is that they are not the same as minerals that already exist in the soil and are sucked up by the plant; they are biologically active compounds created by the plants themselves. Not surprisingly, scientists searching for drugs love them.

Take, for example, my favourite plant compound of the moment: glucosinolate. It's not easy to bring it into conversation—I'm not getting many dates at the moment—but glucosinolate is another substance that our gut bacteria manages to turn into something really useful, a compound called sulforaphane. It doesn't matter if you can't remember the names, the research is amazing.

Firstly, sulforaphane helps rid the body of airborne pollutants. An American university did a study in a town near the Yangtze River delta region of China. They chose it because, unfortunately for the inhabitants, they are guaranteed constant high levels of air pollution all year round. They found that volunteers given a broccoli sprout drink were able to excrete more airborne pollutants than those without. They put this down to glucosinolates and sulforaphane. [98]

So what do you have to eat to get it? It is found in all cruciferous vegetables, but there are particularly high amounts in broccoli, cress, radish, and mustard sprouts.[99] If you're wondering about rapeseed (it is part of the brassica family after all), sadly, it contains far fewer glucosinolates (cancer fighters) than any of its cousins, to the point where some strains contain none whatsoever.[43]

Similarly, it's scary that so many things in the modern world seem to promote cancer, so again it's good to find out that Mother Nature provided her own safety net in the form of other plant chemicals called isothiocyanates. These go around the body mopping up rogue cells before they can proliferate.[100,101]

Where can you get isothiocyanates from? Well, it's those glucosinolates in brassicas again, particularly in the sprouted form.[102] This might be why broccoli sprouts have been shown to reduce nasal inflammation and the risk of flu in smokers.[103] There is evidence that a compound called indol carbol 3 (slightly easier to say), again found in broccoli and cress sprouts but also in all cruciferous vegetables, including mustard greens, can actually convert harsher estrogens in the body to safer ones.[104]

Indole is a fascinating little chemical, which potentially does a lot of good, not least in the prevention of "estrogen-enhanced cancers, including breast, endometrial and cervical." [105] Indoles are linked to bone healing;[106] yet scientists admit they don't know exactly how they are doing it.[107] For our purposes, it doesn't matter how; we just have to eat them up and enjoy the benefits.

Indoles are so good you can buy them as a supplement (£25 a bottle, at the time of writing), and scientists are targeting them as potential anti-cancer drugs.[108,109] Alternatively, grow yourself some mustard, cress, radish, or broccoli sprouts on your windowsill.[102]

So, as you can see, it's important that we eat as many plant hormones and phytochemicals as we can. They help the body balance itself and respond to all the right signals. They top up our hormones or calm them down, whatever is needed. Plus the same plants that are rich in hormones also contain lots of antioxidants, helping flush out any toxins we can't avoid and providing other nutrients to keep our whole system healthy.

In light of all this, it's easy to understand how women in traditional cultures, including our own, who ate diets rich in plant hormones and plant chemicals did not suffer from the menopause symptoms and diseases of aging that are currently rampant in the Western world. Scientists have proved that normal menopause is not about ovarian failure. Healthy women's ovaries will keep working and keep producing the right hormones for us for as long as we need, providing we can get the right messages to and from them. Menopause symptoms are the body's cry for help, telling us that this is not happening. Growing our own plant hormones in the form of beans, seeds, and greens is how we can answer that call.

The pharmaceutical industry, and the supplement makers before them, are looking at plant hormones too. In fact a whole industry is growing up around natural hormones, both estrogen and progesterone, compounded from plants. This is called bio-matching, or BHRT. They refer to the hormones as "bioidentical" because plant hormones have the same molecular structure as our own. Biomatching is very interesting but expensive (see more in Appendix 3).

My problem with BHRT is that they are still trying to isolate, to capture nature's magic, to put it into pills, supplements, and drugs. I think we need the whole plant and all the strange and unfathomable interactions that happen in the body when we eat it, which can't always be pinned down by science.

Plus, there's a lot we don't know, especially about plant progesterone, as the research is very new. It might be that it exerts different strengths in different parts of our bodies, like plant estrogen does. There could be other orphan receptors that look for plant progesterone the way they were found to be looking for plant estrogen. And, not least, there might be other plant compounds that have progesteronic effect apart from kaempferol, apigenin, and diosgenin.

Undoubtedly, scientists will crack it all in the end, and in the meantime, what we must do is eat lots of healthy sprouted foods that have lots of complex phytochemicals, then when the next study comes out showing that some obscure plant compound has amazing effects we can say, "Luckily, I was eating that anyway!"

CHAPTER 7

HOW WE CAN MIMIC TRADITIONAL DIETS IN MODERN WAYS. PRACTICAL SUGGESTIONS BACKED BY SCIENTIFIC RESEARCH

Bill Bryson's book, *At Home*, reports that "The average Londoner in 1851 ate 31.8 pounds of onions as against 13.2 pounds today, consumed over forty pounds of turnips and swedes, compared with 2.3 pounds today, and packed away almost seventy pounds of cabbages per year, as against twenty-one pounds now."[110]

And that's the average Londoner. Mr. Bryson points out that many of the poor lived on bread and water, so that means that the rest of them must have been really going for it.

The problem is that here in the West, nearly all of these types of foods went out of fashion for a long time. Perhaps with the exception of broccoli, the whole brassica family of plants has been struggling to make sales.

Brassica vegetables are also often called cruciferous vegetables, particularly by scientists, and also include bok choy, Brussels sprouts, mustard greens, cresses, cauliflower, kale, cabbage, Chinese cabbage, collard greens, horseradish, kale, kohlrabi, radish, rutabaga, turnip, and watercress. Some are now making a comeback, and restaurants are finding new ways to cook them, but others, such as turnip tops, are no longer even sold by green grocers.

Brassicas contain a whole host of the most wonderful vitamins, minerals, and antioxidants, including all those cancer-fighting chemicals we talked about in the last chapter. The scientists carrying out one study were so impressed by the cancer-fighting ability of brassica vegetables that they concluded that eating high amounts of them is potentially an "effective and acceptable dietary strategy to prevent breast cancer."[104] Another study rightly wondered, though, if it's practical to ask people to eat the amounts of brassicas needed for cancer protection?[111]

This is where sprouted foods come in. Researchers found that, "unexpectedly," broccoli sprouts contain 10–90 times the amount of cancer-fighting chemicals as the full-grown plant. They conclude that "small quantities of crucifer sprouts may protect against the risk of cancer as effectively as much larger quantities of mature vegetables of the same variety."[102]

Sadly, not all brassicas lend themselves to being sprouted without soil, as they come out weedy and sickly, but luckily broccoli, radish, mustard and cress all love it. Eating small amounts of these sprouted foods gives the same benefits as eating large amounts of their mature counterparts, and it means we can mimic traditional diets without having to change our entire lifestyles.

Another investigation into cancer risk found that we need all vegetables, both cooked and raw.[112] While most of us get at least a few cooked vegetables in our diets, we often get very few raw outside of a bit of limp lettuce and a slice of cucumber. So that's another reason to add sprouted foods to our modern diet. They are so easy to eat raw, and you just need small amounts to get huge benefits.

If you're wondering why sprouts are so amazing, it's because they are baby plants that you eat when they are just a few days old and are at their peak of nutrition. The process of germination breaks down nutrients into simple absorbable forms,[113] which has been likened to predigestion[114] as it makes all the goodness more readily available to us.

Another food that sprouting can rapidly turn into a powerhouse of nutrients is legumes or pulses, consisting of beans, peas, and lentils, which were once a much bigger part of our traditional diets than they are for many people today. Humans have been soaking and eating them since Palaeolithic times. Lentils were found in the deepest level of the famous Francheti cave, where Palaeolithic man hung out 13,000 years ago.[115] As we moved forward, lentil dishes became staples in many different cultures. In our own British culture, dishes such as lentils and hock, pease pudding, and spicy lentil soup have now gone out of fashion, which is a shame because they were providing much-needed plant hormones and amino acids.

We need to get these pulses back into our diets. Sprouting makes it easier, because it increases their vitamin and mineral content as well as their digestibility.

We don't have to stick to lentils and peas, either. We can borrow from the Asian traditions and sprout mung beans, either for a few days or grow them to a whole Chinese chow mein–style bean sprout. Sprouted mung beans contain massive amounts of isoflavones, coumestrol, and even lignans, so that's three kinds of plant estrogen.

You also get necessary added fibre from eating these foods, which studies have shown helps rid us of excess estrogen that would otherwise get recycled in the body.[116] Mung bean husks are so wonderful that they have also been studied as an antioxidant in their own right.[117]

For those of you hoping to sprout soya, sadly the beans purchased in the West will not grow the way they do in Asia. This is possibly because the seeds are irradiated to stop bacteria growing, but it stops the bean growing, too. Fortunately, as we have seen, mung and lentil beans more than make up for it.

Possibly the most exciting sprout for the menopausal woman is red clover. As previously mentioned, it has always been part of our folk medicine as well as Chinese and Japanese herbal medicine systems, and even Native American healing traditions.[118] This is not surprising because it contains all three types of isoflavones, including high amounts of coumestrol[119] and kaempferol, too, so that's plant estrogen and progesterone in one handy little sprout.

Its plant cousin, good old alfalfa (sold ready-sprouted in many health food stores, if you don't have time to sprout it yourself) has a similar chemical content, in slightly smaller amounts. One report also noted that it has other very interesting phytochemicals, too, such as carotene, chlorophyll, alkaloids, and saponins.[120]

Don't forget mustard and cress. People are often surprised when I tell them that they are a superfood. While everyone raves about broccoli (including myself, I will admit), they seem to have been consigned to the compost heap of history. Yet a database that listed cruciferous vegetables in order of how many glucosinolates they contain put cress at the top. So in terms of cancer fighting, cress could be even better than broccoli but has none of the kudos.[121]

And finally there's fenugreek, rumoured by herbalists to boost testosterone. Why is testosterone important for girls? For our libidos, for our "joie de vivre," and according to many websites, it will even help boost breast size! A 2015 double-blind placebo controlled study found that it increased sexual desire and arousal.[122] This is no wonder, as we have seen, fenugreek has plant estrogen, plant progesterone, diosgenin, saponins (plant sterols), and apigenin[123] and has long been used for both menstrual problems and menopause problems.[124]

In Part Four (the growing guide) I have listed all of the other reasons you might want to sprout beans or baby greens. This book is about menopause, but the evidence for what sprouted foods can do for other health conditions is so great I had to at least mention it somewhere. This is because sprouted foods are packed with nutrients. So you might, for example, grow mung beans because they contain plant hormones, but you will also be getting vitamins A, B, C, E, folate, calcium, magnesium, phosphorus, potassium, and sodium. You also get trace elements of selenium, copper, and zinc, along with 18 different amino acids.[125]

Sprouting mung beans is cheap and simple to do and makes their nutrients easy for the body to absorb. What's not to like here? Eating sprouted foods is a fantastic way to both mimic those traditional healthy diets and give our bodies the plant hormones we need.

In chapter 6, we discussed the way our own hormones interact with plant hormones and how complex it is, because they all have different strengths and are used in different ways by different parts of our bodies.[126] Nature clearly has her own ways, lots of minute interactions and ways of using all these compounds, and we might never fully understand or be able to mimic artificially.

The bottom line here is that we are trying to keep our ovaries working. Sprouted foods can now be your first line of internal defence, something you are putting into your body to help protect you and your hormone receptors, something that can help you excrete pollutants, something that was always there. Sprouts are the true superfood, and you can get all their wonderful benefits without resorting to the supplements or eating seventy pounds of cabbages a year.

We used to know how to transition through menopause without symptoms, and we can rediscover that. Eating sprouted foods can help us. They are ancient and modern, Eastern and Western.

What's more, we evolved on the kinds of hormones these plants contain. Estrogen and progesterone were around long before us, some 450–500 million years ago, before mammals existed, before there were vertebrates and invertebrates.[127] Animal and plant evolution is so intimately connected that scientists call it co-evolution.[128] They affected us, we affect them. Wild monkeys feast on plant hormones,[129] and we have seen that healthy traditional societies have a bounty of them in their diets. We can also look to our own heritage and see that here, in the West, we ate foods that naturally contained plant hormones and had our own ways of topping them up with hormone-rich sprouts, even herbs. The sad thing is that we didn't know it, so it was easy to push it all aside and call it progress.

Dr. Robert Wilson once called menopause symptoms a hormone deficiency disease, but I believe that many women suffer from *plant hormone* deficiency disease. I do know it's hard to change your diet in this fast food age. That is why sprouting is so exciting.

There are lots of different ways to grow them. Part Four will show you how to find the one that fits your lifestyle. Our bodies need plant hormones. We evolved on them. It's never too late to start bringing them back. You can correct your plant hormone deficiency now. You can *Grow Your Own HRT.*

CHAPTER 8

WHY GROW SPROUTED GREENS AND BEANS AS HRT? IN WHICH, I PUT ALL THAT WE HAVE LEARNT SO FAR INTO HISTORICAL PERSPECTIVE

Menopause symptoms are not the first health problems to be exacerbated by bad diet. One of the most famous is scurvy. It was so rampant during the eighteenth century, it caused more deaths at sea than any other disease, storms, shipwrecks, and even war.[130] Sailors' gums would turn black and spongy, their teeth would fall out, their joints would swell, their skin would blotch, and they would be short of breath before eventually dying an agonizing death.

We now know that scurvy was caused by a lack of fresh fruit and greens, which contain vitamin C. Some people even knew it back then. Apparently, sailors suffering from this terrible disease at sea would commonly "fall upon the greens and grasses of the lands they visited and be cured within days."[131]

Some maritime surgeons and herbalists did use berries, vegetables, and cresses as a cure, but they had to do it under the radar, as the orthodox physicians who held sway at the time had different ideas.[132] Without any maritime experience at all, they surmised that scurvy was caused by anything from laziness, foul vapours, and dampness to blocked perspiration and divine disfavour. They concluded that sailors needed flogging, or poisoning or bleeding; none of it pleasant and none of it worked.[133]

Similarly, menopausal women used to be accused of being depressed, of being afraid of aging, or so spoilt that they had nothing better to do than make up symptoms. Once HRT was invented and big money was involved, then menopause officially became a disease; we were castrates and needed pills and science.

Some brave women have tried to own the situation and say we should embrace hot flushes. They see them as our inner fire and power source, fuelling our rightful anger as women, when all along it was just about a lack of nutrients and plant hormones. How quick we are to attribute the wrong cause when we don't understand things. We just fill the gaps with our big brains and our imaginations.

In the 1800s, the British admiralty certainly fell into this trap. They simply couldn't accept that scurvy was a deficiency disease caused by bad diet. In 1753, a ship's surgeon called James Lind published a book presenting oranges and lemons as the quickest remedy, but no one listened. [134] He wrote at the time, "Some persons cannot be brought to believe that a disease so fatal and so dreaded can be cured and prevented by such easy means."[135] It took another 40 years and many more deaths, before his ideas were implemented.

Here's the really interesting thing. Sprouted mustard and cress can cure scurvy, too. In 1819, when famous Arctic explorer John Parry found his supplies of lemon juice had frozen in the ship's hold during a winter voyage, he turned to mustard and cress seeds that he grew himself in a warm vent in his cabin.[136.] According to one book, "They sprouted and grew in the Arctic darkness, without turning green, and when he fed his ill sailors small salads, those afflicted, had their symptoms disappear."[137]

If they wanted a clue, the nickname for all wild cress is scurvy grass. Yes, scurvy grass. So it's not surprising to find that it's packed with vitamin C (more indeed than can be found in lemons) with an added bonus of other lovely nutrients. In fact, John Wesley's famous medical text *Primitive Physic*, published in 1747[138] (and recently back in print if you want to look it up), pronounces the cure for scurvy as not only lemons but "water and garden cresses, mustard and juice of scurvy grass."

So widely was the cure for scurvy known that most lay medical books written at that time contain references to it. One Polish pastor who lived for some time in England even produced a list of plants that would cure scurvy in order of their effectiveness. Amazingly, without any knowledge of vitamin C or modern testing equipment, he accurately pronounced that cress and scurvy grass were the strongest and most effective against scurvy. He wrote at the time that "the most common herbs and fresh fruits excel the most pompous pharmaceutical preparations."[139]Sadly, instead of being hailed as a hero, he was imprisoned for his religious beliefs and died there in 1742.

Just as scurvy suddenly became an epidemic in the eighteenth century, menopause symptoms are a modern phenomenon stemming from a lack of something in the diet—something we used to eat but no longer do. It is probably more complicated than scurvy, in that the nutritional deficiency is not due to a single essential element missing in the diet, such as vitamin C.

As noted earlier, the first clue that menopause problems are due to diet is that women living in traditional societies on traditional diets, such as the Asian women in Margaret Lock's study, don't get the kind of symptoms and illnesses that Western women do. Furthermore, when Asian women adopt a Western diet, they get menopause symptoms. The next clue is that vegetarian women in Western countries who eat lots of beans and greens also have a less troublesome menopause. So that narrows the search down.

What is it that traditional societies and vegetarians eat in common? The answer is a diet rich in plant hormones—greens, beans, and brassica vegetables.

So far, though, all the evidence is circumstantial; it's just a hunch, taking a punt on the generally available knowledge. And that's all this book would be if it weren't for the many scientific studies on all the different aspects of hormones, plant hormones, and the search for the richest sources of these foods.

Here in the West, some people may think that sprouting beans and seeds is a bit hippy, or something peasants in China and Thailand do. But there are other people seriously into sprouting—white-coated scientists doing controlled experiments in their labs. They extract the rich bounty from sprouted foods to be put into supplements, synthesized into drugs, and sold as a natural alternative to HRT.

This is great, but wouldn't it be better to cut out the middle man, to grow them and eat them ourselves? That's the one thing the studies never say. As a result, we got sidetracked by marketing men, who shoved soya products or plant estrogen supplements on us.

Appendix 2 shows how studies have proven hormone supplements do not achieve the same results as plant hormones that are eaten as part of a healthy diet. The problem is, when the supplements didn't work, people assumed that plant hormones didn't work, so they got sidelined, too.

This is also analogous with scurvy. Our hero James Lind, after producing his book about the lemon cure in the late 1700s, realized that lemons would rot on long sea journeys. So he set about inventing a fruit concentrate by boiling lemons and bottling them. Sadly, cooking the lemons destroyed most of the vitamin C, so when it was tested at sea, it proved not to be as efficacious. This put the whole citrus fruit cure in jeopardy for a long time. That's because boiled lemons, like extracted compounds in supplements, are missing the whole picture.

Lemons were perhaps the soya beans of their day, exotic and foreign. We like the romantic notion of another culture having a special food that can cure all our ills, but the real answer is under our noses. Maybe mustard and cress were too common to be seen as the solution, when in fact, their range of nutrients would have been more beneficial overall than lemons.

Because that's the real question. If John Parry saved his sailors from scurvy by sprouting greens on his Arctic explorations, why hadn't they always done that? Once again, it seems that this knowledge was forgotten. But not everywhere.

As far back as 1598, the Dutch took to growing horseradish and scurvy grass on their ships, in addition to taking along lemon juice.[140] The Chinese always took mung beans to sprout on their sea voyages, which also prevented scurvy, while the Swedish took pine shoots fermented in ale.

Here in England, we also knew about sprouting. A physician called Sir Thomas Browne (1605–1692) mentions it in his book, *The Garden*, in which he explains how to grow cress seeds in water without what he calls "extinction of their general and medical virtues." More specifically, he states that "the seeds of scurvy grass, growing in water pots, have been fruitful on the land."[141]

We used to know how to produce healthy women who could transition to old age without menopause symptoms, and sprouting was part of that. Sadly, it got forgotten, but if you look deeply it was always there, bobbing along in the background, carried forward not just by the hippies of their day but all sorts of people.

James Lind is now famous for being the person the navy should have listened to in 1753, when he promoted his lemon cure. What is lesser known is that nine years later, in his *Essay on Preserving the Health of Seamen*, he discusses sprouting mustard and cresses. He even recommends ways of doing it: "Ships' companies should grow their own salad cress on wet cloths [and] put out blankets in rainy weather to soak the seeds, so that the whole ship, above and below, shall be replete with verger." Verger may be translated as vigour, greenery, or plants; whatever was meant, it's a lovely image.

No doubt some people laughed at this, but in fact, sprouting goes very deep into human prehistory. Before we even started farming, paleolithic people were sprouting wild grains to make bread. This was how they eventually discovered beer and the preservative effects of fermenting! In India, people were sprouting mung beans even before the Chinese. We don't know when we started sprouting mustard and cress here in Europe, but it is there from the moment record keeping began, before the Greeks and Romans even.

Sprouting is part of a long European food culture. It's helped keep us healthy for generations. Yet as we saw in chapter 3, if you go into a supermarket today and buy a little pot of cress salad it will actually be mainly rapeseed. The big suppliers who made this change no doubt found it cheaper this way. What do they care? It looks the same, but as noted earlier, rapeseed has fewer plant hormones, no rich bounty of vitamin C, and more anti nutrients.[142] I doubt that the people who made the swap realized that that simple change would wipe out thousands of years of history.

If it seems strange that the same food that can cure scurvy can also help menopausal symptoms, consider this. Lots of fresh plants have vitamin C and a range of plant hormones; it just happens that sprouted beans and greens are one of the richest sources of vitamins, minerals, and plant hormones on the planet and can in fact help lots of illnesses.

So while lemons were being pushed at sailors for scurvy, the richest source of vitamin C was actually bitter grasses and mustard and cress sprouts.[143] While soya was being marketed to us for its plant estrogen, the biggest source of a range of plant hormones was actually sprouted red clover and mung bean sprouts.

That's the joy of sprouting: lots of nutrients in one place in plants that are cheap, quick to grow, and not dependent on the weather, meaning that sailors can sprout them at sea and women can grow them on their windowsills. I think of sprouting as nature's vitamin pill, a lovely little top-up of nutrients for anyone who wants them.

Some people might think me audacious, comparing solving menopause problems to scurvy. There are probably other analogies, too, because it's a symptom of our human condition—our human endeavour to push ourselves beyond whatever we are naturally able to do. We go on long journeys in massive ships, far away from land. We go to the Arctic. We go into space even. But we return to essential truths—that our fundamental needs as human beings involve good nutrition, plenty of rest, and basic hygiene.

That is the story of menopause, too. We industrialized. We stopped eating whole foods. We processed and refined foods. We tried to bring them back through artificial ways, through drugs and supplements. And now we are faced with the fact that we need ways of getting whole foods back into our diet. Human beings are so clever in what we can achieve, and so stupid in that we keep forgetting the fundamentals.

It's not too late to go back to it all. As a bonus, we now are armed with scientific knowledge, so we know exactly what we are doing. We can borrow from all the different traditions. We can copy the Chinese and sprout mung beans or alfalfa. We can look to folk medicine and grow red clover, mustards, and cresses. We can read scientific studies and grow broccoli sprouts that have really high amounts of cancer-fighting and toxin-clearing chemicals.

Just like those sailors who actually needed even more vitamin C at sea when their bodies were under stress, today we need more plant hormones than ever. We need it to battle all the industrial and chemical hormones in the environment. We need it to make up for the deficiencies in our diets. We need more health-giving properties, not less.

I'm not saying that no-one would have died at sea if they had taken mustard and cress on board, because both supplying and preserving the seed on ships in difficult damp conditions would have been complicated. But it should have been part of the conversation, just like sprouted greens and beans should be part of the menopause conversation, instead of it all being about supplements, pills, or HRT. At the very least, it will help us fill a nutritional gap left when we abandoned our traditional food sources.

If you start growing and eating your own HRT today you will be ingesting a whole host of plant nutrients in their natural form. It's not only the cheap option; it's the easy option. We are going back to something we always did, giving our bodies what they used to have and what our cells have receptors for. Let's not disappoint those cells. Let's get plant hormones into our lives NOW!

PART TWO
– EXPERIENCE –

CHAPTER 9

MY MENOPAUSE DIARY

FEBRUARY 2014

I'm starting this diary because I'm 51, and my periods are getting erratic. Since last year, I've been on an 18–20 day cycle. I seemed to be endlessly "on"—a bit boring when you're looking for a new boyfriend. Whoever said menopause means "men on pause" hasn't met me and my mates. I was quite excited when I had a 40-day cycle. At day 35, I was convinced that it was all over and that my periods had stopped completely. *I have menopaused*, I thought, dramatically (cos I'm a bit like that). I was actually quite relieved that it was all over. The only irritating thing was that I'd just bought a brand new, really large box of tampons!

Before I could give them away, my periods started up again and went back to an 18-day cycle, and with it came waking up sweating in the middle of the night.

I started discussing it with friends.

"Sweats are nothing. I'm soaking the sheets," said one.

"Oh, I'm just hot," I said. "I don't mind. I've spent a lifetime cuddling hot water bottles in bed. I just wish it didn't wake me up at night."

"Go to the doctor and get HRT," whispered another.

"Have you met me?" I replied, pointing to my long, tiered, hippy dress, Birkenstocks, and tray of bean sprouts growing on my windowsill.

"But hippies like you can get the natural alternative to HRT," she replied, "if you go private."

I looked it up online. You can. It's called bio-matching, and it's a mere £800 a year. I noticed in the chemist that they were selling extracts of red clover and soya to help menopause symptoms, but they were £20 for a month's supply.

Then it struck me. I sometimes give talks on growing red clover hydroponically as part of my bean sprouting and baby greens workshop. I have even written a short book on them, and in it, I had noted the estrogenic activity of alfalfa and red clover sprouts. So if they made "natural HRT" by extracting estrogen from these plants, pressing it into pills, and charging a fortune for them, could I achieve the same effect by growing them myself?

It's worth a try.

JUNE 2014

It's four months since I started my experiment. I have been eating red clover sprouts every day, plus mung bean and lentil. I am now on a 23–25-day cycle (and have been for the last three months), and my hot flushes have lessened so significantly that I actually thought they had gone. The weather has just changed, and last night I woke up feeling hot. Is it the weather, or is it me? I honestly can't say yet, but I am keeping tabs on it.

Sprouts surely cannot hold off menopause forever. Just make it easier perhaps? I searched the net for stories of other women eating red clover sprouts. There are none. I searched for the history of red clover. This is more promising. Women have been using it for thousands of years.

I have offered to grow red clover sprouts for my friend Suzi from my meditation group who has terrible night sweats. She said yes, plus I have got another friend called Joanne who is going to grow her own, as she lives too far away for me to grow them for her.

DECEMBER 2014

Ten months since I started taking red clover. I now have no hot flushes whatsoever. We had an Indian summer and warm temperatures right through to the end of October, and I swanned through. I have started reading books on menopause and how menstruating keeps you young, stops your skin from thinning, makes your bones healthy, and slows down aging. I mean, yes purleeeease! I can't believe I was looking forward to menopause. Now I know that I basically want to keep going for as long as possible.

I turned 52 at the beginning of October and was thrilled when the day after my birthday I got my period. *I'm 52 and I'm still menstruating*, I thought. I nearly put it on Facebook. It's a badge of honour now. Plus my periods are now stable again. I am on a short cycle, most months it's 23 days; a couple of times I've gone as far as 26 (and I whooped with joy at the normality). It's so good I'm not yo-yoing like before.

Something else has happened too that I'm almost embarrassed to write about, but don't worry, I'm going to.

Basically, if you read books on female fertility, it will tell you that a sign of ovulation is that we get this clear, jelly like substance. When I was young I had lashings of it. I used to think I had my own KY jelly factory down there. As time went on this declined significantly, and my jelly factory shut down in favour of a more gentle cottage industry. Then as I approached 50, it stopped altogether.

Well guess what? It's back. At the age of 52 and three months, I had a day of jelly. Only one day, but it was enough to show me that my body is still going for it. I honestly wished I had a boyfriend to share it with. But if jelly is a sign of ovulation, I'm wondering, *Could I really be ovulating at my advanced age?* Let's face it, if I got pregnant today, I would give birth just before my 53rd birthday. Surely that would qualify me for the Guinness book of records? All of this is just speculation, of course, but it's exciting, and I'm sure it's all to do with my taking my red clover and other sprouts. Suzi hasn't been back to meditation group, so I haven't been able to test it on her.

JANUARY 2015

I just had a 28-day cycle, followed by a lightish period. Very impressive. It could be that now I'm ovulating again, everything else has fallen into place. I need to know for sure, so I am buying an ovulation test kit online (you get 10 ovulation strips for just £1.99, which seems like a bargain). Women trying to get pregnant use them so they know when to have sex. I hope it comes in a plain bag, else the guy who lives above me will think I'm very odd. He's in his 30s, and I refer to him as "the young man upstairs," as if it is still Victorian times.

So the plan is to wait until I see the jelly and whip out an ovulation stick to find out if it's really happening. I can't wait.

FEBRUARY 2015

I used my ovulation sticks today, and I AM OVULATING. I actually don't quite believe it, so I'm going to do another test next week, late in my cycle, when I definitely can't be. The tests being so cheap, I can do it as often as I like. I am very excited. I feel like I'm a young fertile thing.

END OF FEBRUARY 2015

Just did an ovulation test (knowing I'm due on and can't be ovulating), and it was beautifully negative, so the sticks are real and do work. Also I went to meditation group last night, and Suzi was there. I excitedly told her I'd been growing the HRT and my cycle had evened out and the hot flushes were gone, and she said, "Yeah. Mine have, too!"

I asked, "What are you using?" and she said, "Nothing."

So that means that if I had been growing her the sprouts the way we had planned, we would have thought they were working, when in fact it's all got better on its own. Very interesting. Can't even call it a placebo effect, as she's not taking anything.

MARCH 2015

Last week I missed a few of days of eating my HRT because I went on holiday and got out of the growing cycle. This week I had a couple of mild hot flushes. They woke me up in the middle of the night. I even had to take my bed socks off (lovely image I know). I thought, *Oh the weather has changed, as it's that time of year.* But in the morning, I realized it was still bitter outside, and it must have been me. Luckily, the new batch of sprouts was ready, and it's a few days on now and the flushes have gone.

APRIL 2015

There is not much to report. My cycle for the last three months has been 26, 25, 26, respectively. I'm 52½, and I'm still ovulating apparently. All my friends become wide eyed when I tell them about my days of jelly (or raw egg white as one of them called it, which is just as good a description).

So I was reading part of this book to my writing group (they are all writing very creative novels, sketches, and plays and are very tolerant of me with my menopause book), and as a result have picked up a new client for testing the red clover and mung bean sprouts. Her name is Lisa, and she is starting next week. Another friend from a meditation group called Viryapuspa is having periods that last three weeks at a time! We had a long chat about menopause. She prefers the idea of going to the chemist and buying red clover extracts, but I think I have persuaded her to try growing it as well. In case you're thinking I just talk obsessively to everyone about menopause, I… Oh no, you're right I do!

APRIL 2015

I went for a routine blood test today, and the nurse and I got chatting about menopause. I told her I'm 52 but still menstruating regularly. She said, "Well, I hope you know you still need to use contraception."

I said, "Really? At my age?"

She said, "Oh, yes."

I said, "What's the oldest pregnant women you've known to conceive naturally?"

She said, "Fifty two, but she didn't have any menopause symptoms."

I said, "Nor do I, but I don't have a boyfriend, either."

It didn't matter. She insisted that I took some condoms away with me anyway!

MAY 2, 2015

Just had a 30-day cycle. After months and months of being 25-ish days, I am officially "erratic" again. I have been on one pinch of red clover sprouts a day, plus mung and lentil sprouts, I haven't been on the garlic (which I have discovered also has plant estrogen), though, so will bring that back in and in the meantime, try to eat a tiny bit more red clover.

I had a lovely discovery while researching today. I was writing about all the different kinds of estrogens, and I started to think that we need to separate natural plant estrogens from chemical estrogens. I was thinking, *Dare I be so bold as to rename them?*

It turns out that a very learned man already has (it was buried away in the kind of esteemed journal that I now find myself reading!) He's called Claude Hughes, and the term is *archiestrogens*. It means "ancient estrogens that we co-evolved with." How fantastic is that? I have written more about this in appendix 5. Also I've been reading about monkey diets, and here's the interesting thing: they prefer to eat very young plants. I don't know if that is because of the taste or because they are instinctively drawn to the greater nutrition. But what are sprouts? They are very young plants, which is why I must love them so much.

MAY 8, 2015

Another great day of research. Some days ploughing through scientific papers and trying to understand them is hard. I have spent the whole day reading a paper on plant progesterone, I read the whole thing through three times. Believe me, I usually prefer novels, but this was so outstanding I just had to keep going over it. Every time I went to do something else, I just wanted to get back to reading it! My science teachers at school would be truly astounded.

END OF MAY 2015

I have been writing the section on parabens in cosmetics and what they can do to us and have taken the decision to chuck away my two lipsticks that contain them. I need to throw them out because I honestly can't trust myself, if I'm in a hurry, not to grab one of them and just think, *Sod it!*

So they've gone, and I'm going to invest in some new paraben-free ones to congratulate myself. I also read about the protective power of sprouted foods to shift some of these chemicals out of our bodies. So I gave my sprouts an extra water, and looked at them lovingly.

JUNE 2015

Last month was a 30-day cycle. I haven't been getting the jelly, but I'm not getting hot flushes, either. I have no symptoms whatsoever. Maybe my periods will eventually just stop. I hope so, and I hope that it happens before this book is published, just so that I can report any symptoms.

My cousin Marian told me that she went to 53 before hers stopped, so that might be me, too! I think the lack of jelly is showing me that I am not ovulating. I have decided to start growing fenugreek, as it contains plant sterols and interesting progesteronic compounds, which I probably need. I'm going to see how much I can take every day without taking on its pungent aroma, which has in the past emitted from my armpits!

Or as I like to say: Fenugreek. Don't it reek?

JULY 2015

I just had a 27-day cycle, which is just sooooo normal. Apparently, I can keep menstruating until I'm 55 without officially being a freak, so that's good. Plus all the while I have absolutely no symptoms (though, admittedly, my period was very light). I must be in balance. I have been reading about uterine fibroids (because I have one), and apparently it can up your estrogen levels, which can hold off the menopause. So perhaps that's part of it.

I am taking fenugreek every day now. I read that it enhances the libido. I'll let you know…

JULY 15, 2015

I just stocked up on my supply of paraben-free lipstick. Writing the section on xenestrogens has really spurred me on. However I cannot find a good paraben-free mascara. Sure, they exist, and they look like mascara (which is good because they are expensive), but there's no lash building; they just add a bit of colour to my stumpy lashes. I wouldn't mind that, if the colour could stay put for more than an hour or so. No matter what I do it ends up migrating to just below my lower lashes, giving me that attractive, "I've just had a good cry" look. So I'm back on the old stuff, which probably has parabens, I'm figuring, *It's only on my lashes. How much can they absorb?* I'm telling you this, dear reader, so you know that I have my vanities, too, and you can forgive yourself if you are doing the same.

END OF JULY 2015

Not so good this month. Just had a 22-day cycle, but we just had the hottest day since records began, apparently, and I still didn't get a hot flush, I haven't had one for at least a year. In fact, apart from this short cycle, I don't have any menopause symptoms at all. I should call this My NON-Menopause Diary, about a woman who menstruates normally despite being aging and decrepit in all other respects (yes, some of my back teeth are falling out). Perhaps I am going to sail through to my periods stopping without a symptom (like a good peasant woman living off the land in some remote corner of the globe). Anyway, the hot news is that I've been on fenugreek for about four weeks now. I can't go into detail, but let's say, I'm definitely more libidinous. I'll leave it to your imagination as to what that means.

AUGUST 2015

My period due date came and went without me noticing this month. I was supposed to come on a few days before my holiday and was thinking, *Good. That will get it out the way before I go camping.* I got to day 32 of my cycle, the day of departure. I was packing up my camping stuff and, of course, I came on. Bodies, eh?

Not as bad as a woman I read about in Jenni Murray's menopause book. She went for nearly a year without a period, then booked a romantic break with her husband. Her body clearly thought *I don't think so, dear,* and she came on the day before the flight. So at least my holiday wasn't of the romantic kind. And nor will it be now.

Being late, I am now having the heaviest period for ages. Because of all I now know about menstruation, I'm guessing I didn't ovulate this month, so my womb lining started to build up, hence having a heavier period. Clever, knowing that, aren't I?

SEPTEMBER 2015

Due to holidays, I stopped eating my mung and lentil for a few weeks and then left my red clover out of the fridge, and they went off. As a result, I've been very slightly warm in the night. Very slightly. Plus my periods are officially erratic again. It's day 33 of my cycle, and I seem to have period pains but no period. So I am quickly sprouting another lot. Luckily, mungs only take a few days, and the mild hot flush has gone.

I'm wondering, *Can I take even more plant estrogen?* The monkey studies I've been reading show that sometimes up to 30 percent of their food is estrogenic in any one day, but sometimes as little as 8–10 percent. So I have now decided to grow two trays of red clover a week, rather than one.

OCTOBER 2015

So much for saying it's my NON-menopause diary and talking about my menses being erratic. They are not erratic at all. They have gone, stopped, desisted, ceased. I think, anyway. I have certainly missed a period, and as I turn 53 tomorrow, it seems highly likely that that last heavy period was my last ever period.

OCTOBER 27, 2015

No, they hadn't stopped. A week ago, on what would have been day 57 of my cycle (so almost exactly two 28 day cycles), I came on. It was very light.

NOVEMBER 2015

I was chatting to a woman last night, and when I told her I was writing a book about menopause, she said, "I know everything about the menopause. Mine went on for 10 years. It was a very empowering time."

"Really?" I said.

She explained to me all about "embracing the hot flush" and how the heat is our inner fire and a great chance for women to find their own power.

I must have looked sceptical, because she said, "Have you had hot flushes, dear?"

"Yeah," I said, "but I'm growing plants, and they've gone".

She didn't like that one bit.

"Hot flushes are natural," she said. "They have them all over the world."

I wish I had been gracious at that point. She is a beautiful spiritual woman, but instead, I had to argue and tell her about plant hormones and Asian diets and sprouting.

By this stage we were both almost shouting, which didn't become two middle-aged women at a rather sedate gathering.

Later I thought, *If I'd gone through 10 years of hot flushes, I wouldn't want someone to tell me that I needn't have bothered.* So I will watch that in future.

NOVEMBER 3, 2015

I do so much research online that Google has decided that I am a scientist. It is now showing me pictures of the kind of monkeys and rats it clearly thinks I am experimenting on and offering to sell me the right food to keep them healthy. My dog is appalled! Also it lists a number of hardcore science centres as my eight favourite websites.

Honestly, I hardly know myself anymore. I used to be a stand-up comic—well, 14 years ago. In fact, just before I started all this, I was writing a funny song (I do this occasionally). It was all about middle-aged love and sex and about getting tired halfway through and him not being about to get it up and her having a lack of libido! When I sang it, it got huge laughs, but maybe now I know about fenugreek I can't sing it anymore!

This is my roundabout way of saying I'm still *very* libidinous!

NOVEMBER 27, 2015

I'm having a period roughly every other month. I keep thinking it's all over, but it's forming into a pattern now. I'm menstruating every 40–50 days.

I really think women with a natural lifestyle do have an easier time at menopause. I had lunch with this woman today and inevitably got her to talk about menopause.

She said, "My periods just got lighter and then stopped. No symptoms, nothing." Then she sipped her herb tea and tucked in to her organic flapjack.

DECEMBER 5, 2015

I just had the lightest period ever, and it only lasted two days. I'm calling it a fairy period! I have been compiling lists of foods that contain plant hormones and have worked out that I eat quite a lot of plant estrogens in my diet aside from the sprouted stuff. But here's what's interesting, last week, I came off the red clover and got a mild hot flush. It does seem that red clover is the thing. A friend of mine from meditation group has seen Suzi, and she is having the most terrible time with menopause symptoms now, so maybe she needed the sprouts after all.

JUNE 2016

I haven't written for ages, basically because nothing has happened. I still come on roughly every two months, but each time it gets lighter and lighter. In April, it lasted one day, and a couple of weeks ago it was just half a day and you couldn't really call it a period. I feel that if my menstrual cycle were a song, it would now be on gentle fadeout. Which is surely the way it is meant to be. I have no symptoms whatsoever.

NOVEMBER 2016

I haven't had a period since July. I am now deep into menopause, and my hot flushes have returned. It's only at night, but it's not pleasant. I am eating quite a few sprouts—broccoli, fenugreek, and red clover. I don't have that many sprouted beans, so maybe that's the problem. The hot flushes have horrified me. I started to wonder, *Have I got it all wrong?* So I have decided to take all my own advice. I have upped my red clover to three trays a week and sprinkled slightly more flaxseed on my muesli and completely cut out knowingly eating pesticides.

I buy most of my fruit and veg from my local farmers market, from a farmer who uses minimal spraying. I asked the stall holder which ones had been sprayed, and only bought those that hadn't been sprayed. The farmer looked a bit disappointed. I have been buying there for years. But I have been reading about the "cocktail effect" of pesticides that get in the body. They become part of a toxic stew, and who knows what effects they have? I have had to pay out more for some organic vegetables as a top up, but I feel better about it. If my flushes don't go, I will try taking more mung beans, and if that doesn't work it's supplements for me. At least I'm getting to experiment, I suppose.

DECEMBER 31, 2016

My hot flushes have gone. First of all, they became less intense. I did wonder if it was my imagination, because I won't deny that I want them to go so much. But now they have disappeared, and there is no mistaking that. So I can say it works. Phew!

I am on 100g of sprouted red clover a day, which gives about 40mg of plant estrogen. Strangely, this is the amount they put in most supplements. Plus, as I eat it, I often have a teaspoon of live yoghurt or some sauerkraut for the fermentation.

I am taking linseeds with breakfast but still not having many mung beans at the moment (I think I'm so focused on red clover that I forget about them). I am adding peas and beans to all my dinners. Shepherd's pie with a layer of haricot beans is nice, and lamb and lentil stew equally so; garden peas on days that I don't get any other legumes. It's fairly easy to do.

No period for six months now. Strangely, had a bit of jelly the other day and the libidinousness to go with it! It might be the Christmas holidays or that I'm eating loads of fenugreek. Now, where's that mistletoe?

JANUARY 2017

I now eat so much red clover that I realize why people dry it and use it in herbal medicine or a tincture, it must be easy to just take a tablespoonful. I basically measure it out in the morning and leave it in a bowl in the kitchen so I don't forget to take it. I try to have it before breakfast in the morning, in a salad for lunch, then in a smoothie before my main meal.

I am deeply happy, though, that my hot flushes have gone. I was mortified when they came back, but now I realize that if they hadn't I wouldn't have been able to test my own cure. How I wish I'd known this before. My lovely girls who are experimenting with clover only take one pinch a day. I will let them know as soon as possible that they can take more and tell you how they are doing on my website, along with any new research I find on this subject.

FEBRUARY 2017

Just when I was getting fed up with trying to force beans into my evening meal I have discovered aduki bean brownies. The Japanese have a whole range of cakes made with adukis, because they are the sweetest bean apparently, and slightly creamy too, so lend themselves perfectly to desserts of all kinds. Oh my word, it is delicious and easy to make, so I have added the recipes along with a few others to this book. I'm glad I have discovered this because even though I have got rid of my flushes (again) I seem to be eating unnaturally large amounts of red clover, so if I can get some plant hormones through other means, then all the better. I will keep experimenting with different combinations and put the results on my website. The Japanese also eat aduki beans in a kind of porridge for breakfast, apparently. I was going to try it, but it takes 24 hours to make, and I seem to lack the will to do it. Perhaps it's because I'm so happy with my menopausal muesli blend.

MARCH 2017

The book is nearly done now, I have found a lovely publisher, who does "books to change the world." Next week I'm going to send it off, and it will take on a new life without me. It will go to editors and distributors, and they will take decisions about it. So this is my last diary entry. By the time the book is published, I think I will be officially postmenopausal. It's nine months since I had a period—you have to go a year without a period to qualify.

If you're wondering about the libidinousness: it's still bobbing along in the background! Perhaps it is that the weather is changing, my daffodils are blooming, and the ducks in the park are chasing each other across the ponds. So when the book is done, I'm going to take my trays of sprouts and go on holiday. I bet you'd like to see my diary then!

CHAPTER 10

LISA POPE'S MENOPAUSE STORY

When Sally met me in town during market day and presented me with a green plastic apparatus that I was to sprout my seeds in, I was amused! Would I, the woman who was having nightly sweats, feeling tired and run down, and absolutely hopeless at remembering to take medication on a daily basis, be able to commit to a regime?

Well, yes and no!

I have been able to experience the benefits of red clover sprouting and noticed a dramatic change in my hot flushes subsiding, when religiously eating the natural abundance of, shall we say, "unusual" salad that adorned my plate every day.

However, Sally had chosen someone who gets carried away in health shops and tries all sorts of alternative medicines enthusiastically, then gradually drops them off her morning routine. I am crap at sustaining a health kick.

I am someone who considers herself alternative and have used homeopathy for years, though for some reason I am quite faddish. Well, for the last year, I can honestly say that I have intermittently tried the sprouting of red clover and cress and have really noticed the difference in a short space of time. I can see that when I don't keep up the regime, the hot flushes return and I am as dry as a desert!

Writing this, I feel like I have let Sally down, for not keeping a rigid diary of symptoms and change. But to be honest, it's also quite interesting that I know that I could be making my life less anxious by keeping to the sprouting! So guess what? After letting it lapse for a couple of months, I'm going at it again.

The green apparatus has been cleaned and primed with those precious golden red seeds, and I will be attending to them daily, watching for the growth. I know it will help me fight the flushes and actually put a skip in my step. As I have felt really sluggish, and let's say it out loud, *down* over the last six months.

Perhaps regaining my enthusiasm for sprouting will reboot me, and I will be able to honour Sally's request for keeping a proper diary. I see this more as a menopausal malaise that needs to be shifted and shoved away.

Here is my diary.

DAY / WEEK 1

Feeling bit tired and had restless night… endless flushes… aching joints, ratty, and feeling low.

WEEK 3

I've noticed I've had a change in my vaginal fluids! Yes, jelly-like substance… How peculiar! Flushes subsided slightly.

WEEK 4

Bit more energy. More jelly and ice cream. Flushes fewer. Aching intermittent.

WEEK 5

Same.

WEEK 6 / 7

Oh, dear! Not been disciplined and flushes returned. Took red clover tablets, as travelling about quite a bit. They didn't work as well.

So, in a nutshell: I did notice benefits and changes quite rapidly but needed to keep it going!

CHAPTER 11

KATE TYM'S MENOPAUSE STORY

So here's a snapshot of my life. Married mother of three teenage daughters. I'm 48 years old, generally fit and healthy.

Period wise, I've always suffered from PMT, but it's got more psycho as I've got older and, for the past couple of years, I've had the added delight of night sweats. I am not hot—my temperature is fine—but I am sweating like a racehorse, to the extent that I have to change my nightie as it's too sodden to sleep in. By the time morning comes, I smell like an obese trucker. My periods are horrendously heavy on days 1–2, then peter out. They run over about six days, start to finish.

I would say I approached Sally's sprouting regime with a healthy scepticism, probably in the "Well, I've got nothing to lose" school of thought. I am an exceptionally busy woman. I have launched a new business. I am a writer and performer. I do four cleaning jobs (to bring in income until the business takes off). And I run my house, kids, and husband. So if I can manage to sprout and make a few lifestyle tweaks, anyone can.

After chatting to Sally, I've basically only done the things she suggested that I considered to be easy peasy. They are:

1. Ground up some flaxseed. Sprinkle a good dollop on my muesli every morning.
2. Sprout things. I have no method to my sprouting, just randomly sprout red clover, mung beans, and broccoli, then sprinkle it on whatever I'm having for lunch or dinner.
3. Avocados. I've gone mad for them.
4. No parabens. I'm quite low maintenance in my skin and hair care routine, so I've found it quite easy to just read labels and buy products that are paraben free.

Here's the result. In the times I have stuck to it, I have definitely noticed a change in my psychosis / night sweats. I'm amazed! I have been trying to assess whether the PMT is better or worse (think it's a bit better but harder to quantify as mental rather than physical). Physical symptoms have really improved. When I slack off and don't bother, back they come with a vengeance.

Honestly, the night sweats are horrible, and I can't quite believe things are changing. I've had them for years, then one month of plant munching is making a difference.

Sally persuaded me to keep a diary. Haven't done that since I was a teenager. Plus I'm making nana cake (a bit like banana bread) to keep me off the processed sugary shite.

SAT 12, DEC

Have set up red clover and broccoli sprouts. Have tidied room. Have looked at Nivea body lotion—2 x parabens! Aveeno doesn't seem to have any. Can nick that off youngest daughter as she gets it on prescription (no, that is bad!).

SUN 13, DEC

Dinner: Tonight I made fish stew with garlic, cream, and wine and then I sprinkled some mung beans over mine.

MON 14, DEC

Bought paraben-free moisturizer and body lotion. Sweaty night. Beginning feelings of anxiety. Slight womb ache.

TUES 15, DEC

Ate last of mung beans and Kathy's seeded thins. Sweaty night. Heavy achy womb.

WED 16, DEC

Dinner: smoked trout, salad, bread and pate, sprouted broccoli and red clover. I feel bloated, like if you stuck a pin in me I'd fly around the room. Feel a bit irritable, irrational, fixated.

THURS 17, DEC

A week till Xmas eve! Yay! Santa's bringing me my period for Xmas. Whoop, whoop! Wasn't sweaty last night. Hadn't drank any alcohol (mulled wine doesn't count). Womb achy. Ate a lovely muffin, scrambled egg, bacon, brown sauce, mushrooms, pinch of broccoli sprouts.

FRI 18, DEC

Sweaty night. Slight paranoia/anxiety. Achy womb. Muesli and flax. Cup of tea. Omg! Feel REALLY periody and still four days to go.

SAT 19, DEC

Bit sweaty night. Feel less anxious, but may be masked by feeling hung-over. NOT sweaty in night.

MON 21, DEC

Unsweaty night. What's going on! Feeling pretty normal, which is weird! Having muesli and flax every day. Felt crappy by lunchtime—womb ache and spaced out. Evening: egg mayo, haloumi, beetroot, raw garlic, avocado, sprouts, rocket, 1 x slice bread. Gingerbread from neighbour.

TUES 22, DEC

Really sweaty night. I friggin' stink! Period started, explaining hideous sweatiness! Lunch: homemade pea and ham soup (sprinkled sprouts in it), bread and butter. Evening: made sweet potato curry with spinach (sprouts sprinkled) and rice.

WED 23, DEC

No sweat. Period – HEAVY. Muesli and flax and tea. Lunch: ham sandwich with chutney and sprouts. Evening: stir fry—same as I always do; sprinkled mine with sprouts.

XMAS DAY

All sprouts (except Brussels) were forgotten about!

SAT 26, DEC – SUN 3, JAN

The lost days. Some sprouts, some flax, lots of Xmas cake, several bike rides, out painting and sorting office.

MON 4, JAN

Muesli, flax. Lunch: eggs x 2, avocado, sprouts, brown bread. Evening: pasta, smoked salmon, leeks, cream, parmesan (sprinkled sprouts).

TUES 5, JAN

Muesli, flax. Dinner: pizza with sprouts sprinkled on. Trifle.

THURS 7, JAN

Muesli, flax, and tea. I'm out of sprouts. Waiting for next batch to sprout. My timing was a bit off.

FRI 8, JAN

Muesli and flax and tea. Still feeling normal.

SAT 9, JAN

Bit sweaty night but emotionally normal.

SUN 10, JAN

NOT sweaty

MON 11, JAN

Not sweaty. Sprouts again, so ate last night's curry but with sprouts on it.

TUES 12, JAN

Not sweaty. Ate four choccy biccies (help me, I can't stop!) But had salad with sprouts and 2 x rice cakes.

WED 13, JAN

Feeling relatively normal. Slight womb ache. Salad, avocado, eggs, sprouts.

THURS 15, JAN

Sweaty night. Bit womby, but not feeling mental. Ate omelette, chips, rocket, avocado, sprouts.

FRI 16, JAN

NOT SWEATY. Blimey! Period started two days early. Didn't sleep well but no other symptoms.

SAT 18, JAN

Not sweaty. Instead of muesli, ate porridge with banana, flax, and honey. Lunch: avocado, boiled egg, sprouts, crackers, cheese straws.

SUN 19, JAN

Very sweaty night. I stink. Up at 5.30 to sort out office. Nearly there. Porridge, banana, honey. Need to mill more flax. Evening: cold pheasant and salad and sprouts.

MON 20, JAN

Porridge. Not sweaty at night. Something is working!!

SUN 24, JAN

Muesli and flax. Evening: wraps with salmon and asparagus sprinkled with sprouts.

TUES 26, JAN

Muesli, ground flax, tea. Wrap with avocado, loads of raw garlic for cold, sprouts.

FRI 29, JAN

Muesli. Have gone to spa with Clare!!! No sprouts, as I'm away eating hotel deliciousness.

TUES 2, FEB

Back to routine. Muesli and ground flaxseed. Lunch: salad with chicken, artichoke, beetroot, and sprouts. Tuna, mayo, and sprouts on toast.

WED 3, FEB

Muesli and ground flaxseed. Lunch: meat pie (what??!!) Evening: stir fry.

THURS 4, FEB

Muesli and ground flaxseed. Lunch: two boiled eggs, rocket, sprouts, etc. Evening: wrap with falafel, hummus, rocket, sprouts.

FRI 5, FEB

Muesli and ground flaxseed. Nana cake. Falafel and hummus wrap with sprouts. ½ veg samosa.

SAT 6, FEB

Muesli and ground flaxseed. Bread, pate, and sprouts. Satsuma nana cake. Brazil nuts. Gnocchi and gorgonzola. I've got another cold – arragh! Drown it in two glasses of red wine.

SUN 7, FEB

Muesli and ground flaxseed and nana. No sprouts.

MON 8, FEB

No periody symptoms, but coldy. Muesli, ground flaxseed. No sprouts

TUES 9, FEB

Ate shite all day. Full of cold. No sprouts.

WED 10, FEB

Period started two days early. Is this now a thing? Full of cold. Muesli and linseed. Worst night sweat ever!!!! Gross!!! Still no sprouts, but they are growing again. I'm willing them on.

CHAPTER 12

VIRYAPUSPA NOLAN'S MENOPAUSE STORY

So it all starts in 2013. I have to say, at this point, I'm wondering what all the menopause fuss is about. I have not heard of perimenopause, and really it all seems to be about women unable to come to terms with ageing.

I don't mind getting older, I'm more confident than I've ever been. I don't give a shit about what other people think. I've finally found my look and am living the life I want. I've not put on weight, never wanted or had children, and the sooner my periods stop the better—they have been nothing but an inconvenience and interruption to my life. I have always suffered from very heavy and painful periods, and during 2013, at the age of 46, they are getting lighter and less frequent. Hurrah. If this is menopause, bring it on.

Okay, I realize I have a bit to learn, and it might not be as simple and straightforward as I thought. So I'm now 47, it's 2014, and my menstrual cycle is all over the place. I've started to use the word "erratic." The favourite word of my 15-year-old niece is "random." That seems to sum it up quite well.

Those tell-tale signs of tender breasts that used to signal the onset of my period, giving me a nice weekly warning to prepare myself, has gone. It can be four weeks, two months, three months, and I find myself suddenly being surprised by my period. My body is no longer predictable, and I'm finding it a bit of a challenge. I like order and routine, and this is messing up my habitual way of being.

The real whammy is I'm experiencing severe sinus-type headaches for a day or two during my menstrual cycle. No amount of paracetamol, ibuprofen, steaming, peppermint oil, etc. is having any kind of effect. I have tried to find out if there is any connection to this and menopause, but the Great God Google is failing to come up with any answers.

Right. I'm starting to understand what the fuss is about. So much for my grand plan of simple, no-fuss, period-free, landing into cronehood. January 2015—be careful what you wish for—my desire for regularity has been met. There is however a big BUT. I'm now having a light period every fortnight, two weeks on two weeks off. Er, I was thinking more along the lines of one week on three months off, with a bit of warning, please.

Also I am now learning about the perimenopause, and it's a bit of a depressing read. This is just the start. I am now quite confident that it really is happening, as I've had my first hot flushes, just in bed, and felt them to be quite pleasant really—just a warm glow doing a Mexican wave up my body. Then I started getting hot during the day. The odd one or two flushes were quite manageable, but this then became hourly alongside untreatable sinus migraine, the whole thing lasting for two days. Great!

My partner Paris then got chatting to Sally, provoked by the comment of a bell-ringing chum. "Oh, the menopause. Whatever you've been through so far in your relationship, you just need to be really understanding and patient."

Next time I see Sally, she pounces. "You need to take red clover," she says.

She was a convert and actually was the sole source of information as to what is causing the headaches. It's estrogen, apparently. It's my body's way of saying, "Drop an egg." As they are now a scarce commodity, nothing happens. So it sends a bit more estrogen—nothing, as it continues to pump in the hormone. The result is hot flushes and headaches. I now know why, so now I need to stop it.

The quickest way is to head off to Boots the Chemist and grab red clover tablets. They are staggeringly expensive, and if this process is years rather than months, I'd be wise to buy some shares in the company. However, I am desperate.

It is now March, and the fortnightly cycle is wearing a bit thin. After two weeks of taking the tablets, the flushes have ceased. So has the fortnightly period. Hurrah.

March 2015. Sally rolls up with seeds and a sprouter, tells me about the red clover sprouting process and how much to take. I'm not one of life's natural sprouters, despite being into the Buddhist vegetarian thing. I find it easier to buy things in packets from Marks and Sparks.

I sprinkled and watered. They burst into life, and I got a bit excited. I forgot to water a few times and have a few false starts.

There is a certain discipline required. It would be safe to say that my house plants thrive on neglect. The same is not true of a sprout seed. I usually remember to sprinkle water on at breakfast and forget later on in the day. I then find myself looking at a tray of dried seed. There is something of a Lazarus quality about the seeds, though, as they seem to be miraculously revived when watered again and crop quite well, despite a day or two of lying dried out and dormant. This is rather a good job, as I work away from home two days a week, and my beloved partner is equally negligent and watering can be a bit sporadic.

I have to say sprouting is not that travel friendly, and I have now got the knack of harvesting a crop and putting it in the fridge in sealed Tupperware, where it seems to stay quite fresh for about a week. Though due to working away and periods travelling away from home, it is not always possible/practical for me to take it in plant form.

I have to say, I rather lack Sally's enthusiasm for sprouting, despite the benefits. I'm obviously not a natural gardener. I have not got the knack for timing, so I either have sprouts or don't and have to grab a tablet instead. I'm sure there is a timing thing of sowing, growing, and harvesting, but my rather hectic life and poor menopausal memory rather makes this a hit-or-miss affair.

However, despite being a reluctant sprouter, I find it quite easy to grow on the whole, and there is something satisfying about having something green fresh and living on the kitchen window sill. I feel rather smug that it gives the illusion of living a healthy back-to-nature life when people come round. Before you know it, I may be making raw chocolate and having turmeric lattes.

I'm in a routine of consuming a generous pinch per day, usually at breakfast, and continue with a tablet, which I take in the evening. I nervously ate my first pinch, expecting it to taste disgusting—things that are good for you traditionally aren't that tasty. To my surprise, it just tastes a bit like bitter lettuce. I've not discovered any amazing recipes, and as it's not highly flavoured, it can't really be added to things as a herb. So beyond just sprinkling some on the odd salad, I tend to just stand at the fridge and grab a pinch.

In April and May 2015, I experience no flushes or migraine. Oh yes I've got this nailed. Then it seems to be either feast or famine.

In June 2015, great joy: the period that lasted 21 days with headaches but no flushes.

July and August 2015: no period, flushes, or migraine. Perhaps that three-week one was the finale. Perhaps it's now all over.

It's not! I'm going on retreat for two weeks in Spain. It requires plane, train, bus, and a 40 minute trip in a 4WD to get there, so packing seeds and sprouter is out. I'll just take the tablet form, which will be a good experiment to see if it's really working. Yep, it's working

September 2015: I just take the tablets and have a two-day migraine. Once I return to the UK, out comes the trusted sprouter, and I am once again seeding, watering, and sprouting.

October 2015: no period, flushes, or migraine.

November 2015: had period, no flushes, or migraine.

December 2015: had period, no flushes, or migraine.

January to March 2016: no period, flushes, or migraine. I am a red clover convert, and I have everything crossed that this is it. Bye bye period, hello menopause. Generally, I take the plant form five days out of seven, and also take the tablets. It's become my security blanket. I fear to stop it, in case I get a blasted headache.

April 2016: changed brand of red clover tablet from Menopace to Holland & Barrett. They are cheaper; they are 2-for-1 in their penny sale. Surely, they are all just the same, right? During April, start to have flushes, no migraine.

Beginning April: Noooo! I have a period but no migraine. I am still sprouting.

May 2015: life was just too busy. I work away from home a bit. I had been on retreat for five days. The consequence of all this: I had no plant form of red clover for two weeks. Due to age and the fact that my memory no longer seems to work, I had no tablet form for three days.

The result: I begin to have hourly flushes for a two-week period and suffer two migraines. At least, no period. The flushes, though, are dreadful. It's not just that I feel hot or have a "tropical moment"; I feel like I'm coming down with flu. Sometimes I'm wondering, *Is this a flush, or am I ill?* I have to say, there seems to be a bit of a conspiracy of silence on this. Trying to work it out. Trying to find out the symptoms of perimenopause seems to be like trying to find out about the black arts—actually, that's probably easier.

They say ask your mum. Mine seems to be very vague (*Oh, it took about a year. I didn't really notice it*). My mum is not the most self-aware person, and I'm sceptical. My sister, who lived at home during that time, in response to my question said, "She was a complete cow."

So at least the good news is I'm not noticing any mood swings, and my partner has not noticed me growing udders or having a tendency to moo.

I've changed back to Menopace red clover tablets and am now regularly sprouting. Flushes and migraine ceased in mid June. So currently no period, flushes, or migraine for three months. I'm always hopeful this will be the end, but it isn't.

I had a period in August. I thought, at least one period every three months isn't bad, though it seems to come with an accompanying side dish of untreatable two-day migraines, even if taking plant form.

The up side is they seem to be more regulated, I'm not having flushes or migraines between periods. My moods seem okay. I'm not randomly bursting into tears or having angry rages.

I had three periods in December, January, and February, then two months of hot flush sinus/migraine hell. I realized that when I run out of red clover in plant form (when I'm away and can't grow it), the supplement doesn't seem to have any effect on its own. So I decided to up the dose of sprouted red clover to two or three pinches a day. I'm pleased to say I'm now back to being flush free. So when Sally wrote to say that she's been experimenting, and that I should increase my dose to three large pinches a day, I was able to tell her I already had!

I have to say that, despite my poor growing skills and non-conducive life-style, I do feel that I have a greater sense of well-being when I'm eating the sprouts and seem to enjoy good health and energy. Which is encouraging me to sprout a bit more, rather than relying on tablet form, which is rather against the grain. I am much more a quick and convenient sort of a woman.

I'm now 49—three years into perimenopause, the whole process being a whole lot more than I had bargained for. I continue to have everything crossed that this will be my last period.

CHAPTER 13

Joanne Edward's Menopause Story

I peer at two trays slotting nicely on top of one another, the top one an array of small, bright green clusters of tiny plants. I normally can't grow things. They wilt as soon as they look at me. But red clover is very, very easy. Swamp it in water in the tray twice a day, drain it, and it'll grow in a week. Amazing.

I really need to grow it, as my hot flushes are serious. It starts as a solid mass, shoots into my head, and crashes into my skull. A surge of heat fires up and down my back several times, and water starts to seep across my forehead and my upper lip. My heart bangs against my chest at such a rate that my hands are shaking to keep up. The heat seeps up from my spine onto my face, and I think I can only have become the red of a furnace.

I always feel like this will never stop and then suddenly the heat begins to subside, to be replaced by a spawning kind of sickness and deep shock. So as you can see I needed to do something. And being a bit alternative I try this first.

The first time I grow them I actually hurry home from work to look at my seeds. They were lying in the tray, which I had watered and drained, as instructed. Out of the sides of most of them, a small white bud was beginning to push.

"You're growing," I say. It's a first.

The shoots then became stalks, bendy and springy and kind of enthusiastic. A bit like me, I think. I haven't felt this enthusiastic about something for a while. And I'm not bendy, not any more. I am achey and stiff and very, very tense. It feels like PMT, only this PMT has lasted 12 tetchy weeks. I've not had a period in four months.

The stalks then sprout small, green, proud leaves. I was quite liberal with the seeds, so the tray is packed quite tight, adding to the excitement. I couldn't wait. I wrenched some green sprouts out of the tray and put them into my mouth: a strange, sweet, unaccountable euphoria sweeps through me, and I try some more. I start putting clover in everything. I put it in salads and sandwiches, and I try it in cakes and on my cereal.

I can't quite put my finger on it—though I frequently do, plunging my index into the springy mass of shoots growing on the tray—but there is something cheerful about these little plants. Is it just because I am enjoying growing them, or is it because for the first time in years some of the spots scattered over my face are retreating, and this would make any acne sufferer happy.

Or is this cheery feeling not just about being able to grow a plant, but actually what that plant could be doing for me? Is that possible? Something so tiny, so green, so easily grown could do so much? A happy hormone?

Sally has talked me into eating less sugar, too, and that is helping. Everything seems to be going well until I get this terrible, terrible cold. Every bit of me above my shoulders feels swollen.

"I thought they were stuffed with vitamins, these plants. I shouldn't be like this," I tell Sally.

"They are—vitamins and plant hormones—but they're not magic," she says. "Having a cold is no reason to give up."

But I do give up.

It's like I have to stop taking the plants to see the full evidence of their influence. I stop for a while, and my stomach becomes a great, hard barrel; my forehead, an acre of furrows of worry scattered with spots; my knees, unbendable; and yes, I have my first almighty rush of heat and downpour of sweat in months. I fish out the seeds, and they sound like rain as I pour them onto the tray.

I stick at it this time.

I start to notice the elasticity about my body, my skin, like it's stretchier instead of tense. I will never be able to bend like I used to be able to do, but the sense of being a ramrod permanently on the verge of breaking has stopped. And I wait and wait for the hot flushes, like a victim under siege. And those hot flushes don't come.

Sally is right: they're no miracle, these little green shoots; they are just practically, solidly good.

I still have spots, I just don't have new ones every week, and sometimes they fade, whereas before they just grew ever more furious. I still have new aches that I don't think will go away, but I can work with them, instead of being stuck under or with them. I still put on weight but it's not an unmoveable, solid, sore weight. And, most extraordinary, somehow, because so very unexpected, I still have periods; intermittent, light, infrequent periods but, nevertheless, strong, brilliant reminders that I am older, but not yet old, old. I never thought I'd be happy to have a period, but somehow I am.

I talk to the plants and tell them how great they are doing. They manage, in their resilient, clambering way, to look pleased.

I don't know why they feel like friends instead of just plants. It must be because there is something very alive about what they do for mc, and because I have, in a way, built up a relationship with red clover—from my reluctant start to my excited loved-up middle to my mature and grateful now.

PART THREE
– APPLICATION –

HOW MUCH DO I NEED TO TAKE?
HOW MUCH AM I GETTING ALREADY?

I hope what you have read so far has convinced you to grow your own HRT. If so the next thing you will quite rightly want to know is, "How much do I have to take?"

I'm going to suggest we all increase the amount of plant hormones in our diets to match those of countries who have fewer menopause symptoms.

The first thing you need to work out is how many plant hormones you are getting in your normal diet. Appendices 7 and 8 are databases of foods that are high in plant estrogen and progesterone, so you can find out the specifics. But below is a general guide.

Let's start with the most famous plant estrogen, isoflavones. These are found in high amounts in nearly all beans, including runner beans, green beans, mung beans, chickpeas, and lentils. Most nuts and seeds have reasonable amounts, too. If you're worried that you're not eating many of these foods, you're not alone: American women eat an average of 1.54 mg of isoflavones a day, whereas the Japanese get 40 mg.[144, 145]

If you don't like beans it's not a problem, because traditionally Europeans got lots of their plant estrogen from lignans. These are found in nearly all fruits and vegetables, especially linseeds, sesame seeds, dates, apricots, avocados, garlic, broccoli, prunes, and chestnuts. Swedish women (who also have fewer menopause symptoms) get an average of 16 mg lignans a day, whereas in the UK it's 1 mg. [146, 147]

The strongest yet least known plant estrogen is coumestrol. There are small amounts in many fruits and vegetables, but to get it in concentrated form you need to eat sprouted mung beans, alfalfa, or red clover. Korean women, who eat a lot of sprouted foods and get few menopause symptoms, eat an average of 30 ug of coumestrol a day, while American women get

0.6 ug.[148, 149] The same sprouted foods that contain coumestrol contain lignans and isoflavones too, so you can see that they can really help you top up all of your plant hormones.

The figures above are just averages, because amounts vary drastically (Japanese women actually eat 20–80 mg plant estrogen a day). So we don't have to get hung up on exact amounts; we can start small and build up to what works for us. I started off with one small pinch of red clover a day, then went up to two, and finally three large pinches when I became seriously menopausal (see my diary for more on this). For the record, a 6-inch (15cm) tray of red clover, grown to double leaf stage, weighs 130–140 g, so a large pinch is roughly 20g of red clover, or 15mg of phytoestrogen (plant estrogen). This is interesting because most plant estrogen supplements offer 20–40 mg a day.

Of course, what really matters when we are growing our own HRT is the *effect* plants have on us, not what's in them. One study has looked into this and measured the estrogenic impact of a number of contenders.[150] Guess which came out top? Soya? Red clover? Neither. It was kudzu root, which is native to Asia, and sadly we can't grow it on our windowsills. Luckily, close behind was red clover blossom and red clover sprouts. Next came mung bean sprouts, then alfalfa sprouts, followed by green beans and soya beans. It really was a joy to see this study, with all the sprouted foods holding their own.

As for plant progesterone, we saw in Part One, scientists have only recently proven that compounds such as kaempferol and apigenin are converted into it by our gut bacteria.

For this reason, there are no estimates of what traditional societies are eating. When the late Dr. John Lee prescribed progesterone cream, he recommended 15–30 mg a day, so that's worth aiming for. Plant progesterone is more concentrated than plant estrogens.

The top foods for plant progesterone are capers, cumin, parsley, raw garden cress, raw broccoli, raw watercress, garlic, raw gooseberries, raw strawberries, and raw apricots. If eating this kind of food is a problem, I'm sure you know what I am going to suggest the answer is: sprouting, of course. Radish and fenugreek are the top progesteronic sprouts, but all the brassicas are good.

CHAPTER 15

ALL OF THE SYMPTOMS AND MORE!

So now you know roughly how many plant hormones are in your diet, the next thing you need to think about is your symptoms. At the end of the day, feeling well and healthy is what this is all about.

I accept that some women might have very serious long-term or genetic problems with their ovaries. If you have severe symptoms, unusual bleeding, or pain, you should always consult your doctor. Most of us have been watching our own cycles since puberty and know roughly what is going on.

Below is a chart which shows how each sprouted food can help with our hormonal balance, prevention of illnesses, and also particular issues. Underneath, I have gone into more detail about each condition, for those who need to know more.

If you really want to find out if you are producing sufficient hormones, see if you can get your GP to arrange for you to have a blood test. If you have cash to spare, you can buy tests online or consult a nutritionist. Normally, the test consists of taking saliva samples over 11 days that monitor both your estrogen and progesterone levels.

WHAT SPROUTS CAN DO FOR YOU

Issue	First Choice	Other Choices
Fertile women with long cycles and heavy periods (non-ovulation)	Mung beans	Beans, radish, cress, broccoli, and other brassicas
Perimenopausal hot flushes	Red clover	Mung beans or flaxseed
Headaches	Red clover	Any of the brassicas
Postmenopausal	Radish or cress and one of the beans	Any sprouted foods

Issue	First Choice	Other Choices
Dryness, vaginal atrophy (too little estrogen)	Red clover	Fenugreek
Baldness/hair on chin (too much testosterone)	Flaxseed	Broccoli or radish
Lack of libido (too little testosterone)	Fenugreek	Flaxseed
Cancer prevention	Broccoli, Cress or Flax	All Sprouted greens are associated with cancer prevention, particularly brassicas
If you have had or are at risk of hormone- dependent cancer	Flaxseed	Red clover
Osteoporosis prevention	Red clover, cress	Radish, or any brassica
Heart health	Aduki, mung beans, or try alfalfa (for high choles-terol)	Any beans will help
Withdrawing from HRT	Mung beans and cress	Any estrogenic sprout, especially red clover
Multiple orgasms (sadly not guaranteed!)	Fenugreek	Flaxseed

FERTILE WOMEN/NON-OVULATION/ TOO MUCH ESTROGEN

If you are having long cycles followed by heavy periods, there's a good chance you are not ovulating. If you want to know for sure, you can normally tell as your fluid becomes clear and jellylike around day 12 of your cycle. If that is too icky to contemplate, you can buy ovulation sticks that you pee on, which tell you within 10 minutes whether you are ovulating or not.

If you find that you're not ovulating, it most likely means that the problem is with your ovaries or the signals they receive. The upshot is that you won't be producing much progesterone, which makes you estrogen dominant. Bean sprouts such as mung are perfect for this. You can't go wrong, really, because, as we saw in Part One, plant estrogens act as a top-up when we don't have enough estrogen and as a calmer when we do.

The other reason to focus on sprouted beans is they contain fibre that helps the body get rid of excess estrogen.[151] Plant estrogens also help the liver produce SHBG (sex hormone binding globulin). I've mentioned it before but just to remind you: SHBG binds to our hormones and excretes them from the body.[152] So that's one sprout, three different functions.

You will need to grow something progesteronic to balance it. We have seen that cress, radish, and fenugreek contain high amounts of progesteronic compounds and are a lovely garnish too. If you don't want to grow more than one sprout, then try red clover, fenugreek, or alfalfa, as they contain a good combination of plant estrogen and progesterone, although in different concentrations (red clover has more).

You also need to look at why your ovaries are not receiving the right messages to enable them to ovulate. One big reason could be your exposure to EDCs in the environment (see chapter 17 on how to avoid them). If none of this works, you will need to consult a specialist. Do try this first, though, as it certainly worked for me. Natural foods rich in plant hormones will help get the body healthy again so that it can do what it is meant to.

PERIMENOPAUSAL HOT FLUSHES

The most discussed sign of being menopausal is hot flushes. They can vary from a gentle warmth enveloping our bodies to a wild-and-crazy, soaking-our–sheets-in-sweat-and-running-out-into-the-snow type of thing. Part One explains that hot flushes are a side effect of our ovaries not doing what the hormones produced in our brain via the HPA axis have asked them to do.

The absolutely best sprout for this is red clover. Not only has it been used for thousands of years to cure all sorts of menstrual problems but the science behind it is stunning. Red clover gives us all of the different plant estrogens, including coumestrol, which helps calm down those brain hormones, plus plant progesterone.[153]

Its plant cousin alfalfa also has a broad range of plant hormones but in smaller amounts. You may have to grow and eat more to get the desired effect, but alfalfa is easier to source. Mung beans also contain large amounts of coumestrol, and studies have shown that flaxseeds have a distinct effect on menopause symptoms.[154]

So you have lots of choice on this. Go for what fits into your life or the sprouts you most enjoy growing.

Headaches

A less obvious sign of perimenopause is increased headaches or migraines. John Lee, MD, explains that estrogen imbalance causes our blood vessels to dilate and this, along with water retention, can bring on cyclical migraine, usually just before we menstruate. He argues that headaches are a classic symptom of estrogen dominance.[155] All of the plants mentioned above will help: mung beans, red clover, and alfalfa. Dr. Lee thought that progesterone helps fight migraines, so try radish, mustard, cress, and broccoli sprouts if migraines are an issue for you. Any of the tangy brassicas will do (refer to Appendix 7 for progesteronic foods). Viryapuspa's diary in Part Two talks about her experience of this issue.

Postmenopausal Women

When we go through menopause, our ovaries stop making estrogen and progesterone but still make male hormones such as testosterone, which our fat and muscle cells convert into estrogen. In this way, postmenopausal women still make as much as 60 percent of the estrogen that a fertile woman does. Our ovaries also stop making progesterone after menopause, but the adrenal glands will make us a small amount. The adrenals are fascinating little glands, which sit on top of the kidneys, and are responsible for making 50 important hormones, including those for regulating sex hormones and stress, so if we are under stress, then production of progesterone is affected.[156]

In traditional societies, it's likely that older women rely on plant progesterone to keep their bones strong and their systems healthy, and we can too. Try any of the brassica sprouts, such as radish, broccoli, mustard, or cress, or even mix a few of them together. They are all wonderful general tonics for the older woman.

Even though we don't need as much progesterone once we go through menopause (no more womb monitoring for it to do), this precious hormone is still essential for the healthy functioning of the central nervous system, the brain, for bone building, and estrogen clearing, so do take this issue seriously.

Vaginal Atrophy / Dryness (Too Little Estrogen)

Dryness where we were once so juicy, and no energy to have sex, even if we fancied it, is often the first sign of low estrogen levels and can occur at any time. More serious symptoms are vaginal atrophy (shrinking of the vagina, causing sex to be painful), vaginismus (tightening of the vaginal muscles), and feeling the need to pee all the time.

Plant hormones can help, and researchers have been putting them to the test. A study specifically looked at genistein (an estrogenic compound found in red clover) and observed that it had good effects on the vaginal tract.[157]

So if you are in this situation, definitely grow red clover or alfalfa sprouts (lots of them), and if you can add some sprouted beans, such as mung beans, all the better. This will help boost your plant estrogen levels.

Interestingly enough, unless you are very slim, most women are more likely to be estrogen dominant. This is because, as mentioned above, fat and muscle tissues also convert other hormones into estrogen. So if you are lacking estrogen, it might be that you need to look at your overall health, liver function, and toxin load to find out why.

If your symptoms are extreme I would go to the doctor, because if you don't sort out vaginal atrophy, in particular, it can have long-term consequences. Depending on where you live there are different things the doctor can prescribe. In the UK and Asia you will be offered estriol cream (estriol is the special older women's estrogen good for vaginas that I mentioned earlier). You use it topically, and it plumps up the vaginal wall without causing problems elsewhere.[158] Estriol cream is not available in the US, (I have explained why in Appendix 3); instead, you will be offered creams containing estradiol.

A 2009 review of the evidence on this subject concluded that if you are postmenopausal and have vaginal and lower urinary tract symptoms, using estrogen cream "can offer significant benefit with low risk." [159] This is the nearest I come to recommending traditional HRT. You can get it from your doctor, or there are a number of creams you can buy online, or you can go the alternative route and buy plant hormone cream.

HAIRY CHIN AND MALE PATTERN BALDNESS (TOO MUCH TESTOSTERONE)

We all get a bit hairier than we'd like as we get older, but hirsuitism (thick manlike hair on the face) combined with male pattern baldness (losing hair on the crown) is another matter. It's generally accepted that these conditions are linked to too much testosterone.

In a healthy person, testosterone levels are kept down by compounds such as sex hormone binding globulin (SHBG), which not only stops testosterone from attaching to our hormone receptors but escorts it from our bodies. Therefore increasing our SHBG naturally is a good idea, and phytoestrogens such as those found in sprouted mung beans and lentils will do the job.[160] Eating flaxseeds specifically has been show to reduce hormone levels in patients with hirsuitism (and polycystic ovaries, for that matter).[161] This is to do with flaxseed's high phytoestrogenic content, plus they contain fibre, which we have seen is another way of helping the body eliminate hormones efficiently.[162]

It's long been known that hirsuitism is linked to weight gain, insulin resistance, and polycystic ovaries, which again are all connected to liver health.[163] See Chapter 16 (and your doctor) if you think you have liver problems.

If you are postmenopausal and get a sudden onset of hirsuitism, it could be linked to ovarian or adrenal tumours, so do get it checked out. [164]

Lack of Libido
(Too Little Testosterone)

Lack of libido, depression, tiredness, and memory lapses often go together. If you are suffering from any of these, the first thing to do is have your iron and thyroid checked, as low levels can be a major cause of this, too. If these levels are okay, and you are producing enough estrogen and progesterone (have a hormone test if you're not sure), then it could be that you have too little testosterone.

The theory that lack of libido is caused by low testosterone levels is based on the fact that fertile women get a testosterone peak around the time of ovulation; it might be that this gives us that extra nudge to procreate. Women who have had their ovaries removed commonly suffer from lack of libido, even though they are being supplemented with estrogen, so clearly it is something else they are missing. A number of studies have treated women suffering from low libido with testosterone. Some results were very encouraging,[165] but overall, the results are inconclusive and more research is called for. [166]

It's important to note that all of the studies on testosterone supplementation used synthetic (man-made) testosterone not bioidentical testosterone, which is identical to the testosterone your own body makes. It's a much better idea to look at why our bodies are not creating enough testosterone in the first place, and try to increase it naturally. Ideally, what we want is the perfect amount of testosterone that gives us great libido but doesn't lead to masculinizing effects.

This is where fenugreek steps into the limelight! Two recent studies on fenugreek supplements, both of them double blind and placebo controlled, show that fenugreek can increase levels of testosterone in the body and sexual desire in women.[167] A study of men found the same, and in particular, noted an increase in morning erections![168]

We have already seen that fenugreek is very special because it contains diosgenin, which is usually associated with wild yams and used to create progesterone supplements in the lab. What is less known is that diosgenin can also raise DHEA (dehydroepiandrosterone), the hormone precursor to testosterone in the body, along with its estrogenic properties.[169] That's a powerful punch for one little plant.

Diosgenin is found in greatest amounts in the young leaves and mature seeds of fenugreek.[170] The reason to go the sprouting/young leaf route is that as already noted, the unsprouted seeds contain anti-nutrients, which can lead to digestive troubles and gas. Sprouting them to double-leaf stage is quite easy, too.

If you can't bear fenugreek (some people can't), try flaxseeds instead. Although the main claim to fame of flax is the high amount of plant lignans it contains, what is less well known is that flaxseeds contain lots of interesting plant sterols too.[171] Dr. Lee certainly thought that plant sterols play a part in hormone production, and while I couldn't find any human studies, male water buffalo in India that were fed flaxseed showed increased libido and semen quality.[172]

Finally, there is a case to be made that the libido side of things can be due to having the wrong partner, and I'm afraid not even sprouts can cure you of that! A study entitled "Sexual satisfaction in the seventh decade of life" found that relationship satisfaction was strongly linked to sexual satisfaction.[173] If you think this is really your problem, you might want to try the other kind of HRT—Husband Replacement Therapy. Apparently, it is very popular amongst baby boomers and has few side effects!

CANCER PREVENTION

I have already talked about this subject in earlier parts of this book, but here I'm going to bring together all my evidence about sprouted foods and cancer prevention in one place. The link between cancer prevention and diet is so great that if you type those two words into any science website, you'll be offered thousands of research papers. When it comes to cancer prevention, brassica vegetables generally, and sprouting in particular, come into their own.[174] There are 54 studies just on broccoli sprouts and cancer alone.

The reason is that lots of cancers are linked to hormone imbalance in both men and women. Estrogen is active throughout the body, where it encourages cells to divide and grow. Without the right balances, this can lead to cancer.

Sprouted plant foods can help. As noted earlier, if we have too much estrogen, plant hormones will fight to get on the receptors on our cells and offer incredibly weak doses of hormones to calm everything down. Brassica sprouts also have compounds called indoles, which help convert harsher estrogens linked with increased risk of cancer, to weaker ones.[104]

This alone would be reason enough to eat broccoli, cress, radish, or mustard sprouts, but brassicas also help our bodies make a compound called sulforaphane, which assists with getting rid of toxins and harmful chemicals from the body.[175] This could be why one study concluded that cruciferous vegetables might "slow, halt, or regress" the progression of both tumours and blood cancers.[176]

The next thing you need to know is sulforaphane attacks tumour stemness,[177] this is the ability that cancer cells have to keep growing indefinitely, rather than die naturally, the way normal cells do. You can see why scientists like these compounds and are keen to find out how they work.

One study followed sulforaphane through the digestive tract and found that it was active in the stomach and liver but got to other organs in much lower doses.[178] However, other scientists have found that even a single dose of broccoli sprout preparation became measurable in human breast tissue.[179]

This might be because, as we have seen, sprouted brassicas contain 10–90 percent more glucosinolates (the precursor of sulforaphane and indoles) than full-grown vegetables. They also contain a compound called myrosinase (more about this later) which helps convert those lovely cancer-fighting compounds into their active form. Studies have found that the presence of myrosinase made sprouted broccoli seven times more effective than supplements. [180,181]

This is all so exciting that it is attracting mainstream attention. "How Broccoli Can Help Fight Cancer," announced a Daily Mail headline recently.[182] For me, what was really amazing is that the paper printed a picture of a plate of broccoli sprouts. The article noted that the race is on now to make a "broccoli pill" to be used in new drugs that can halt, cure, or prevent cancer.[183]

But until they do, we have to keep eating the real thing. If you're wondering how much you need to eat for cancer prevention, it seems that anything you can do will help. One population study (where they track the diets of people over several years) found that having more than one serving of brassica vegetables per week led to fewer cancers.[184] Another study suggested that five servings of cruciferous vegetables a week or taking broccoli sprout extract would do the trick.[175]

For our purposes, an American study found that a single dose of 68g of broccoli sprouts had significant anti-cancer activity in both the prostate and colon.[185] Whilst these studies focus on broccoli, don't forget that cress is just as rich in glucosinolates (the precursor to sulforaphane) but doesn't get the same attention. So sprout some brassicas today, and get yourself some cancer prevention.

REPRODUCTIVE AND HORMONE-DEPENDENT CANCERS

The big question I get asked is whether eating plant estrogens is a problem for women who have had, or are at risk of developing, hormone-dependent cancers. This is where the cancer cells themselves have hormone receptors and are looking for hormones to land on them to help them grow.

First, the good news is that plant hormones eaten as part of your diet have always been linked to a much reduced risk of all cancers, including those that are hormone dependent, to the point where they can be seen as a preventative.[186] So that means you can eat all your hormone-rich beans, peas, and seeds to ease your menopause symptoms without worrying.

In fact, consumption of plant estrogens such as lignans is associated with reduced risks for both estrogen- and progesterone-dependent cancers. [44, 187] This is true of postmenopausal breast cancer, too.[188] So it's worth reminding you again that flaxseeds contain the highest amount of lignans of any plant and that they have been proven to inhibit hormone-dependent cancers.[189]

Consuming 24g of flaxseeds daily for four weeks actually shrank breast tumours,[190] and in the petri dish, sprouted flaxseeds killed human breast cancer cells[191] (which doesn't mean that they can do that in our bodies, but it's a start). Another study looking specifically at lignans found the fibre they contain might be having an impact on breast cancer survival.[192]

Flax is one of the few seeds that if you can't sprout, you'd be wise to just grind it up and eat it anyway. Just don't buy supplements.

Cancer websites, such as Oncologynutrition.com, advise their readers that dietary plant estrogens are okay, and you can take 2–3 tablespoons of ground flaxseed a day. However, they do suggest that if you have had a hormone-dependent cancer, you should talk to your doctor, dietician, and health care team about adding flaxseeds to your diet.[193]

Unsprouted flaxseeds do contain anti-nutrients, which is why it is best to at least soak them overnight. If you get fed up with flaxseeds, try increasing your sesame seed intake, as they are the next highest source of lignans and have the added bonus that they make nice desserts and biscuits.

All of the brassica sprouts contain lignans, too, so that's yet another reason to start sprouting them.

The next big thing that I get asked about is women who have already had hormone-dependent cancers and now take tamoxifen. This is a drug that blocks our hormone receptors so that hormones cannot land on them and promote growth. The problem is that we do need some estrogen, so not surprisingly tamoxifen has side effects. The most common are hot flushes, fatigue, mood swings, depression, headache, hair thinning, constipation, dry skin, and loss of libido, which, of course, are all the same as those associated with women having a bad menopause.

So do plant hormones help or hinder? So far, one rat study has found that red clover does not interfere with tamoxifen in rats or in human liver cells;[194] a full human study hasn't taken place yet, but it looks promising. Flaxseeds have been shown to work with tamoxifen to fight breast cancer, which is exciting.[195, 196] The reason to take plant hormones whilst you are on hormone-blocking drugs is that our plant hormone receptors may work differently, and this could be a way of getting some of the safe, gentle hormones that you are missing.

This also holds true of aromatase inhibitors. These are often given to postmenopausal women with breast cancer as it stops us from converting the male hormones that our ovaries naturally produce into estrogens.

Not surprisingly some of the side effects of blocking this action are the same as those of too much testosterone: aggressive behaviour and hair loss, along with osteoporosis and liver dysfunction. Again, plant hormones can help. Flaxseeds have been found not to interfere with the drug; in fact, it was the other way round: the aromatase inhibitor reduced the amount of circulating lignans.[197]

Secondly, plant hormones themselves act as weak aromatase inhibitors.[198] For these reasons, large-scale studies are being called for to see how they can fit into overall breast cancer strategy.

Plant hormones are obviously only part of the solution, but if you want to know the link between diet generally and breast cancer specifically, it's this: a study published in 2016 followed nearly 50,000 Japanese women for 14 years. Those with a Westernized diet had a 32 percent increase in breast cancer overall, with postmenopausal women having a 29 percent higher chance of getting cancer than women on a Japanese diet. The most startling conclusion was that those with an "extreme" intake of Western food had an 83 percent higher risk of breast cancer.[199]

This doesn't mean we all have to eat a Japanese diet. We have our own healthy traditions we can turn to—whole, fresh foods and salads rather than the denatured, nutrient-free, processed offerings that are sadly considered to be a modern Western diet.

OSTEOPOROSIS PREVENTION

Estrogen and progesterone play a huge role in what is called bone turnover and renewal. Estrogen is in charge of finding weak points in our bones and removing them, leaving little tiny holes. Progesterone then comes along and fills them in with new bone. Osteoporosis develops when the two hormones get out of balance, and you have too many holes left unfilled. The bones eventually become so porous that they become fragile and break more easily.

Brittle bone, on the other hand, occurs when we lack estrogen to scavenge out the old bone in the first place. In the short term that is okay, but it means that bone never gets renewed and slowly deteriorates, becoming weaker, brittle, and thus more liable to break.

Sprouted foods can help because of their rich bounty of plant hormones and other flavonoids that scientists know help bone renewal, formation, and mineralization.[200]

We have already seen that plant estrogen helps balance our hormones. A 2003 review of 43 different studies concluded that, "eating foods rich in phytoestrogens has bone-sparing effects in the long term."[201]

A number of rat experiments have shown that red clover is especially good for bone health,[202, 203, 204] and helps increase mineral absorption too.[205] A 12-week, double-blind, placebo-controlled study in which women were given a red clover extract that had been fermented with lactic acid bacteria reported that bone mineral density increased.[206] This is interesting, not just because of the fermentation element but because the whole plant was fermented rather than just consisting of extracted isoflavones. This means that the participants would have benefited from lots of other plant nutrients, not least plant progesterone, which offers a wonderful top-up for postmenopausal women who might otherwise lack it.

The other great sprouts for osteoporosis are all the brassicas, including cress and radish. They contain really high amounts of kaempferol and apigenin, and have been long associated with strong bone formation, even before we knew they were progesteronic.[207, 208,209]

In fact, so many studies showed that cress is good for fracture healing,[210] healthy bones, and bone turnover, it prompted a clinical trial looking at cress's potential to heal osteoarthritis.[211] Ninety-eight patients with osteoarthritis were given 6 grams of powdered cress daily for 30 days. Amazingly, 30 percent of patients went into complete remission, another 37.5 percent of patients showed marked improvement, and 25 percent moderately improved. Only 7.5 percent patients received no relief at all.

Plant hormones are not the whole story, though. One of the biggest promoters of good bone health is any kind of exercise, especially weight-bearing exercise.[212] I'm sure you have all heard of Dowager's hump. It's where osteoporosis causes you to have a strange curvature of the spine, an unsightly hump at the base of the neck and a stoop. It is so named because dowagers (titled widows) would have been particularly susceptible to developing the condition, having so many servants to do their lifting and carrying for them.

Since I have found this out, I think of every activity as "bone building," from carrying my shopping in a rucksack to putting the rubbish out. I even clean my flat with a bit more vigour, thinking to myself that it's doing me good.

The next important thing to remember is that hormones are really the messengers. Without the right vitamins and minerals to carry out the actions, such as vitamin D, calcium, magnesium, and zinc, we will still be at risk. The wonderful thing is that there is another old-fashioned remedy for this, and that is to eat ground-up egg shells and make your own mineral mix (see Chapter 18 for more.)

It's never too late to start looking after your bones. They constantly change and renew. If you are in any doubt about how your bones are doing, ask your doctor for a test, especially if you are postmenopausal and have a family history of osteoporosis.

HEART HEALTH

Beans and legumes of all kinds have always been associated with heart health. This is because they are a wonderfully low-fat source of protein and have ample vitamins, lots of lovely fibre, and phytonutrients. A Canadian team reviewed 26 different randomized trials and concluded that just one cup of legumes a day is associated with lowering LDL cholesterols and less risk of heart attacks.[213]

Some people do worry that legumes also contain the anti-nutrients we talked about earlier in this book. I expect by now you know what I am going to suggest—yes, we need to sprout them. Sprouting sloughs off anti-nutrients and increases fibre, vitamins, and phytonutrients. How can you say no?

All sprouted beans are good. Aduki beans seem to be the most studied in terms of impact on the heart and circulation. Researchers report that they can reduce hypertension,[214] regulate glucose tolerance,[215] and excitingly, are a natural anti-obesity agent.[216, 217]

Mung beans give them a run for their money, though. The Chinese have done a lot of research into them and into what one study calls the "dynamic changes" during the sprouting process.[218] This is what turns a plain old bean into an antioxidant, antimicrobial, anti-inflammatory, and anti-diabetic powerhouse. Beans are so associated with heart health that I would say that even if you never sprout a single one, you should still eat them. Cooking reduces the anti-nutrients slightly, but if the thought of being a bit windy is putting you off, a very serious study called "Perceptions of flatulence from bean consumption," done by Arizona State University, found that under 50 percent of people reported flatulence whilst eating half a cup of baked beans a day, and that went down to 19 percent for black-eyed peas.[219] I was very excited by this and tried eating them myself and, sadly, found them no less fartworthy than other beans!

It's fairly easy to get legumes into your life. Chapter 18 will show you how.

If for any reason you absolutely hate beans, then the good news is that lignans are also associated with heart health. This is partly to do with the fact that all the same things that are rich in lignans, such as flaxseeds and vegetables, are also full of fibre, but one study managed to separate the two things and found that even lignans alone had an impact.[220] This means that sprouted flax and fenugreek, any of the brassicas, and red clover will all help heart health, or to put it more simply, *any* sprout. You have no excuses!

IF YOU ARE ALREADY ON HRT

If you are worried about the health risks of being on HRT, the good thing is it's never too late to change. Valerie Beral, one of the authors of the Million Women study, when interviewed, said that, "Once you stop taking HRT, the risks start to melt away."[221]

Current NHS advice on HRT is that if it is used on a short-term basis (no more than five years), the benefits outweigh the risks for women with menopause symptoms.[222] However many studies have shown that using HRT for over 10 years increases the risk of breast and endometrial cancers, as well as heart disease (see Appendix 1 for more on this).

If you want to come off of HRT and are worried about how to go about it, the answer is that you should reduce it slowly with the help of your GP. The great news is that you can start taking plant estrogens and progesterones while you are still on it. Natural plant estrogens pose no danger when consumed as part of your diet.

Have a look at the estrogenic foods in Appendix 7, and get yourself into a good bean habit. Start sprouting mung and cress, as they are easy and between them will give you a good range of hormones. If you are feeling ambitious red clover is the most wonderful hormonal plant. The plant hormones will challenge the synthetic estrogen getting on your receptors and weaken its impact.

If you are taken off HRT suddenly, you might want to use plant estrogen supplements whilst you learn to start growing sprouts, and perhaps adjust your diet, as it's not easy to change overnight,(see Appendix 2 for more about taking supplements).

AND FINALLY ... HOW TO HAVE MULTIPLE ORGASMS

Having more than one orgasm cascading through a sex session is actually more likely for an older woman than a younger one. How fabulous is that? Some postmenopausal women have been surprised by their sudden ability to have the multiple orgasms that have eluded them all their lives.

Dr. Debby Herbenick, of the University of Indiana, says that orgasm becomes easier with age. She found that whilst 61 percent of women ages 18 to 24 experienced orgasm, a massive 70 percent of women in their 40s and 50s did.[223] She argues that it is because we are more relaxed, we know what we like, and we are prepared to ask for it.

There could be another explanation though. Reduction in estrogen means our testosterone, which has always been there, gets more of a chance to work its magic. Testosterone makes you randy, basically. Female to male transsexuals who start having testosterone injections often report (with shock) how they suddenly can't stop thinking about sex.

Don't be afraid of testosterone, though; it's all about balance! The advice I gave in the section above on how to avoid problems with libido is the same way to have a fantastic postmenopausal sex life.

All the plant hormones and complex plant nutrients that you are growing in little trays on your windowsill will help with libido, but if you really want to go for it, then you need to start growing fenugreek.[224] As previously mentioned, the problem with eating the seeds alone is that it can lead to you smelling of them. The sprouts are much gentler, and if you can pick ALL the seeds off individually you can largely avoid it. Yes, it sounds like a hassle, but when you feel the effect rippling through your nether regions you might find it's worth it.

If you need an incentive to try and get your libido going again, it's this: we've got to use it or lose it. Sex (even on our own) helps keep vaginal muscles healthy. They need exercising, like every other part of our bodies. So come on, girls, make the most of it.

Later-life divorce is rapidly on the rise in both Britain and America, yet interestingly, so is later-life marriage. This means that we are not getting divorced to live lonely, sexless lives with our cats, but in order to find someone more compatible with whom we can have great sex.

Don't worry if you don't always fancy it. Just make the best of it when you do. A study of older women in California found that even though they had sex less often, they reported deeper satisfaction from orgasm.[225]

The researchers found that the ability to enjoy sex was not about age but about general health and feeling well, which is a good lesson for us all.

This is our heritage as older women. We evolved in order to make society richer, deeper, and to pass on knowledge. None of this is unique to humans. Older postmenopausal killer whales not only lead the pod and know where to find food in times of famine, they also have sex with the younger males. Deborah Giles from the Centre for Whale Research thinks that this is to "teach them sex education." [226] It could just be recreational, though. Maybe those younger males worship their leader. Maybe it's bonding. Who knows? But it all looks like fun.

CHAPTER 16

WHAT CAN YOU DO IF IT DOESN'T WORK?

If you have trays of red clover on your windowsill, mung beans growing in bags above your sink, if you're putting linseeds on your breakfast, garnishing all your meals with sprouted broccoli or cress, and having avocado and garlic with your salad everyday, and you are still struggling with hot flushes, poor libido, or dryness, this chapter is for you.

INCREASING YOUR GUT BACTERIA

I have mentioned this a few times, but it's worth saying again. It's gut bacteria that turn all the plant compounds we have been talking about—the isoflavones, lignans, and coumestrol—into plant hormones.

The number of illnesses linked to a lack of gut bacteria is astounding. It's not just the obvious ones like Crohn's disease and irritable bowel syndrome that are impacted, but obesity, diabetes, multiple sclerosis, arthritis, and, of course, menopause symptoms! No wonder The British Medical Journal has called gut bacteria, or the microbiome, to give it its proper name, "the new frontier in science."[227]

How do you know if you have enough of the right gut bacteria? If you have taken a lot of antibiotics in your life, and particularly in the last year, then you probably won't have. If you have any autoimmune illness, then you're unlikely to have a healthy gut, either. Scientists are starting to realize that some of their studies into foods and health are skewed by subjects not having the correct balance of gut bacteria.

Live probiotic yoghurts can help. A study from the University of London found that many contain the bacteria they claimed on the label and that these survived in the gut for longer than probiotics sold in solid form.[228] They also found that probiotics are best taken on an empty stomach (which is a shame because I've been eating yoghurt as a dessert for years).

The bad news is that commercially available products often only offer a few strains of bacteria which might not be enough if you have a serious problem. There is another solution. If you're going to grow your own HRT, why not ferment your own gut bacteria, too? It's another thing that traditional societies do naturally.

Europeans have sauerkraut made from salted cabbage, the Japanese have tempeh, natto, and miso made from fermented soya beans—many societies, including our own, used to ferment vegetables such as onions and beets to make old-fashioned chutneys. Before refrigeration was invented, we had to do this so that we had food in the winter.

The right bacteria not only stops food from going off but also actually enhances it by giving us lots of lovely probiotics. But many of the things we used to ferment naturally, such as cucumbers and eggs, using no additives except salt, are now preserved in harsh vinegar, which kills both good and bad bacteria.

You can still buy traditional sauerkraut and other fermented foods. Look down what my friend Chris lovingly calls the "weird aisle" of your local supermarket, or go to a health food store. Sauerkraut has a long history of keeping us healthy. Captain Cook famously took it on his sea voyages and kept his sailors healthy. If you are taking plant hormone supplements then look for ones that include gut bacteria in the formula (see Appendix 2 for more on supplements), or eat them with probiotic yoghurt.

The Role of Prebiotics

If you are going to go to a lot of effort to get probiotics into your life (and tummy), you need to make sure they survive and proliferate. For this we must eat what are called prebiotics. This was a fairly new word to me until recently, and now it seems to be everywhere. Basically *pre*biotics feed the *pro*biotics.[229]

Good prebiotics include all raw vegetables, especially Jerusalem artichokes, leeks, onions, and garlic.[230] The diets of all traditional societies contain a certain amount of raw food, and we should carry on that tradition; a bit of lettuce in your burger is not enough. The wonderful thing, of course, is that you can eat your sprouted foods raw. How about a salad every lunchtime? Or a green smoothie once a day? Or a raw garnish on every meal. Find a way to get that raw veg into your lives, and it will repay you in so many ways.

HOW TO MAKE SURE YOU GET ENOUGH MYROSINASE

Obviously sprouted foods are not just full of wonderful plant hormones but also cancer-fighting chemicals, known as glucosinolates. We have already seen that it is gut bacteria again that turns them into their active form sulforaphane, but here's the exciting thing: chopping, juicing, or chewing your vegetables releases a substance called myrosinase, which will do the job, too.

Myrosinase is very spicy, which explains the high amounts in radish, mustard, broccoli and particularly cress.[231] [232]

Lack of myrosinase is another reason supplements do not always work as well. A study specifically compared eating broccoli pills with broccoli sprouts and found that the pill takers were unable to convert them to sulforaphane.[233] Another study found that broccoli powder didn't contain sulforaphane, but air-dried broccoli sprouts did. If subjects ate them both, the sprouts helped convert the powder to sulforaphane as well.[234]

Cooking destroys myrosinase, but steaming is better; [235] however, to get the maximum, you need good bacteria and myrosinase. It's interesting that there are high amounts of myrosinase in mustard. So all those centuries when people mixed mustard and cress, they couldn't have known that they were combining a plant with the highest amount of glucosinolates with a plant with the highest amount of myrosinase, yet somehow they just knew it was healthy. How very, very clever of them.

MAKE SURE YOUR LIVER FUNCTION IS OKAY

When I talked earlier about estriol, the special older women's estrogen that is good for hair, skin, and vaginas, I mentioned that it is converted from other hormones by the liver. If we have too many hormones floating around our system, it is the liver that breaks them down for excretion. If we need to convert harsh estrogens to less harmful ones, yes, it's the liver again. Scientists are also now thinking that the liver's role in hormonal balance is so important that it can protect us from breast cancer.[236]

So what upsets our livers? The good news is that it's the same old stuff that upsets the rest of our bodies, so it provides more reasons to do the right thing, rather than another new set of rules to worry about. Yes, it's processed foods, chemicals from the environment such as pesticides and plastics, and, of course, good old drugs and alcohol.

The liver is actually marvellous in that it can handle a certain amount of these things, and it's the only one of our organs that can regenerate itself, but it needs the right tools. It uses nutrients to process hormones and bile to excrete them. A paper written by the Women's International Pharmacy likens the liver to a sewage works. It says that if you don't have the right nutrients, then it's like not having enough sewage staff. This can cause toxins to build up and leak back into our bodies which can lead to illness.[237]

So what are those nutrients?

The liver likes all the basic vitamins: the B group, including B12, and C and E. It also wants things you might not have heard of, such as calcium-D-glucarate, sulphur, glutathione, and methionine. But don't worry: these are all found in fruits and vegetables, egg yolks, fish, and meat.

If you are eating a reasonable diet, you should have enough. If not, you might want to consider taking supplements, but here's the rub: some supplements can cause liver damage.[238] Not all of them, obviously, and more research has been called for, but I would look for supplements that don't have chemical coating and fillers—so that's the expensive ones![239]

Finally, what your liver needs is to produce bile, which escorts all the nasty things we put into our bodies out again. If you think you're short of bile, then common old dandelions are known to increase it by up to 50 percent. One study's authors were so impressed they suggested that this humble weed be a potential therapy for patients with acute liver disease.[240]

It's very easy to add dandelions to your smoothie everyday. Young ones are especially good, but if you don't want to crawl around your garden looking for them, there are dandelion supplements or you can sip dandelion tea.

Liver function is an important subject. If you suspect something is wrong (and we have already looked at hirsuitism), you'd do well to have it checked out because the liver has so many functions in the body. I have just picked out those to do with hormones, but basically, as many alcoholics have found out, if we keep abusing our livers, we die.

WHAT IF YOU REALLY CAN'T EAT HEALTHILY?

I'm guessing that a lot of people reading a book called *Grow Your Own HRT* will already be fairly healthy eaters. The big question is this: if you're living on pizza, chocolate biscuits, and ice-cream, is there any point in trying to grow your own HRT?

The answer is YES! It will help, but it won't solve all your problems.

Sprouted foods have tons of vitamins and trace elements that you might be missing, plus the plant hormones. Sprouted food also helps the body to detoxify. So if you can add sprouts to your pizza, it's something, it's a start, it's cheap and easy, and nutritious, and the mere fact that you are doing something for yourself is marvellous.

As ancient as sprouting is, as a concept it feels like a modern, fast, easy way to maximize the potential of vegetables. Some studies are calling sprouts "functional foods." This means that they are more than just nutrition; they have specific jobs to do in the body and might help end the degenerative problems that are called "Western Diseases."[241, 242]

So just do what you can do. Nudge yourself in the right direction. Always make the slightly better choice. If you're vegetarian living on processed foods, move to lovely, old-fashioned bean stews and spicy lentil soups. If you're a meat eater, try fresh meat recipes rather than the processed kind and have lots of vegetable dishes with it. Just keep trying. Everything you do can help. Some people eat healthily in the week and allow themselves to pig out at weekends. Others go on the 5:2 diet (*The Fast Diet*) and actually semi-fast for two days a week and eat what they like the rest of the time.

Don't beat yourself up about it. Just do what you can when you can. Grow a little tray of sprouts on your windowsill, and let them tempt you into eating them, every day.

EAT A WIDE VARIETY OF FOODS

This whole book is based on current scientific understanding, but intrepid scientists keep finding new compounds, new interactions, and new things that we need in our diets. I've been writing this book for three years, and I can barely keep up. I've been banging on about the three major kinds of plant estrogens, but science is discovering more all the time.[243]

For example, studies of sesame seeds found they are just as good as flax-seeds in terms of estrogenic impact, but the scientists have yet to identify how they are doing it.[244] We have seen that red clover is more progesteronic than it should be, according to what it contains. There is so much more to be discovered.

We've talked about plant estrogen and the recent discovery of plant progesterone; next, I think plant testosterone will be proven to exist, too! I would be willing to bet that it's in fenugreek—studies are already showing that some of the compounds it contains bind to testosterone receptors.[245]

Secondly, as complicated as this book may seem, I have been keeping it simple. The scientific studies it is based on are far more detailed than the way I have described them. Compounds such as isoflavones break down into a number of other compounds, which scientists test and break down into more minute particles.

This is why we must try to mimic what our ancestors ate, because there are interactions among plant compounds that we probably can't even imagine yet. Scientists think that as we were evolving, there were masses of plant chemicals washing through our systems. So never dismiss any vegetable, especially if it is local and easy to grow; you never know what it might be doing for you. Current thinking is that we should "eat the rainbow" on our plate at every meal, because plant nutrients come in many different colours, each with their own special attributes, making sure we have a bit of each is a great way of ensuring a balanced diet.

Don't deny your body its heritage. Don't just eat what's fashionable. Give your body what it needs, and it will reward you many times over.

Synthetic Hormones, Chemical Hormones. What Are They? Where Are They? And Why You Should Avoid Them

There is a great deal of evidence that chemical estrogens in the environment interfere with our reproductive organs.[246] News stories often focus on their effects on infertility,[247] but we older women still need our ovaries, too, in order to stay strong and healthy.

A recent American study looked at 31,000 women whose bodies had high levels of hormone-mimicking chemicals, known as endocrine disruptors, and found that they were going through menopause 1.9 years to 3.8 years earlier than those with lower levels.[248] The researchers noted that early decline in ovarian function could increase infertility, heart problems, osteoporosis, and other medical problems. I can't imagine having an early menopause because you are so full of toxins is a pleasant experience, so here is my guide on how to avoid them.

Synthetic Estrogens in Cosmetics and Toiletries (Known As Parabens)

We love our creams, potions, and lotions. We douse ourselves in them, bathe in them, spray them on, rub them in, and make sure they are really absorbed into our skin, yet many of them contain parabens that could really harm us.

Parabens hit the headlines in 2004 when researchers found them in breast cancer tissue samples.[249] Some companies immediately took them out of their products, whilst others argued that just because parabens were found in tumours it didn't mean that they had caused them; they might just be stored there.

It's a fair point, and research is now showing that in isolation and at low doses, *some* parabens might be fairly harmless, but others are not. It's the accumulation of them in the body that causes problems, even at levels previously considered safe.[250]

Fortunately, the European Union is on this. It has limited the total amount of parabens in each product to 0.19 percent. Sadly, it didn't ban methylparaben, which is one of the most popular cosmetic preservatives. A 2016 study has shown that methylparaben helps breast cancers grow AND helps the malignant cells resist cancer treatment, not a good combination.[251] This is why commentators like Marilyn Glenville, PhD, a leading nutritionist, psychologist, and author, argue that we should particularly avoid rubbing creams containing methylparabens into our breasts.[252]

In the United States, there is no current ban on any parabens in cosmetics and toiletries, but a number of companies are producing paraben-free cosmetics, all over the world, so we can all avoid them if we want to.

Which Cosmetics and Toiletries Have Parabens?

To find out if your favourite product contains parabens, just look at the label, and it should tell you. Companies are legally obliged to list their ingredients, although you may need a magnifying glass to read them.

The major ones are:

- methylparaben
- ethylparaben
- isobutylparaben
- propylparaben
  (just as you're probably getting the idea that they handily say "paraben" here's a few that don't):
- hydroxybenzoic acid
- hydroxybenzoate

The EU has completely banned five parabens from toiletries. These are:

- isopropylparaben
- isobutylparaben

- phenylparaben
- benzylparaben
- pentylparaben

Two international brands that I was surprised to see still use parabens are the Simple range and the Body Shop.

The Simple website states uncategorically that parabens are safe and are indeed best for people with sensitive skin.[253] They provide a link to a 2007 EU directive to prove this. I think they are assuming people won't bother to read it, and I might not have myself, if it were not for writing this book.

However I followed that link and read it (in full!), and I'm glad I did. EU Directive No. 1223/2009 (oh yes, I'm getting sexy now) makes quite chilling reading. It bans some parabens, notes the hormone-disrupting effect of others, states that parabens try to attach to human estrogen receptor cells, and calls for more research. This is why, as mentioned previously, from 2015, the products themselves have to have maximum levels of 0.19 percent parabens.

The Simple website further justifies including parabens by saying, "Although the commercially available product is produced synthetically, parabens do occur naturally in plants and animals."

So their argument is that because estrogen occurs naturally, it's okay to put synthetic estrogens in cosmetics. Really? That's like saying, "Although this blow-up dolly is made of plastic, natural females do exist, so she is a proper girlfriend. Honest."

WHICH COSMETICS DON'T HAVE PARABENS?

All organic cosmetics and toiletries are paraben free. Be careful of products that say they are "natural," because that term is meaningless. To qualify as "natural," a product just has to have something in the mix that was natural at some stage.

A number of high street brands are paraben free, including:
- Nivea Pure & Natural range
- Palmers range of cocoa butter products
- Clinique have changed their formulation of Dramatically Different Moisturizing lotion and created Dramatically Different Moisturizing Lotion Plus, which is paraben free.
- Aqueous cream from BP doesn't use them.

- Beauty Without Cruelty was the original anti-animal testing cosmetic company and does not contain parabens (or palm oil, for that matter).
- B range from Superdrug (UK only)
- CVS (USA only) has a list of 58 paraben-free products on its website.

For a complete list of paraben-free cosmetics and toiletries, go to the website of Breast Cancer Action. They keep an up-to-date list of all paraben- free brands and invite companies to write in with their status. And by the way, their website is unequivocal that parabens increase the risk of breast cancer. See more at *www.bcaction.org/our-take-on-breast-cancer/environment/ safe-cosmetics/paraben-free-cosmetics*

SYNTHETIC ESTROGEN IN WATER

Firstly, the good news is that British and American tap water is the safest and cleanest in the world, with regulatory bodies making sure it stays that way. The bad news is that if you live in a building with old pipes or bad water mains, it could add contaminants and bacteria on the way.[254, 255]

That's mainly bacterial, though; it's the chemicals and hormones that might affect our reproductive systems that we are interested in.

British water companies are not obliged to carry out tests for estrogens in the water they supply, but those that do, state that the levels are so low as to be undetectable. Again, this sounds good until you find out that male fish have been turned into females in water that had synthetic estrogen at levels as low as one part per billion, which qualifies as undetectable.[256]

So it's powerful stuff—for fish, anyway.

For us, we do know that more men are growing moobs (man boobs), and fertility is declining, but that could be due to all sorts of chemical and environmental pressures, of which water is only one factor.[257] We also know that when fish are affected by estrogens in the water, it does pass up the food chain, which eventually means us.[258]

Some sources say that you can avoid estrogen in drinking water by using a simple water filter, but I can't find any hard science behind that claim. I know some people find water filters just too fiddly to muck about with, and some people can't remember when to change them. (I always do it on the first of the month, as that way I never forget.)

There are lots of other reasons to use a water filter, as they get rid of contaminants like mercury, so it really is just a case of doing our best. If you are rich, there are lots of other water filtering systems, such as reverse osmosis. These involve plumbers and take up space, but they do get rid of estrogens in the water. Meanwhile, the race is on amongst scientists to create a cheap, easy, biofilter with organisms that will eat their way through anything nasty in the water. I'm really looking forward to that happening.

HORMONES IN FOOD

There's lots you can do to avoid eating synthetic hormones in food. The first thing is to go organic. If you can't afford that, try local farmers markets and farms that use more traditional farming methods, such as crop rotation, minimal spraying, and respect for the environment. Prices are usually as cheap as the supermarket because you're cutting out the middle man, and you are getting lovely local food. You can also get weekly veggie boxes delivered to your home, or become friends with your local allotment growers, who often have a surplus.

If that is impossible, wash your fruit and vegetables carefully. Some websites say you should peel them; others say that there are antioxidants in the skin that will help the body rid itself of pesticides! I couldn't find any definitive studies saying which is best.

If you eat meat and live in Europe, growth hormones have been banned for some time, and the EU has stopped imports of meat containing them. This has upset American ranchers who still routinely use growth hormones, and a battle has been raging ever since.

American consumers are starting to demand fewer growth hormones now, though. One article in the *Huffington Post* asks "Have you ever noticed how much bigger some U.S. cows, chickens, and turkeys are than their European counterparts?" and goes on to list all the things allowed in American food that are not allowed on European plates.[259] Growth hormones in food are causing lots of worries, not least that children are reaching puberty much earlier, although the culprit is not just growth hormones but, interestingly enough, eating refined sugar.[260]

Some companies are starting to respond. In 2015, McDonalds stopped using milk from cows treated with growth hormones in their milkshakes. So there is hope that many companies will respond to consumer pressure and that we are all heading in the right direction.

Synthetic Estrogen in Plastics

The research into synthetic estrogen in plastics is really quite frightening, but it's been known for a long time, and there is lots of legislation in place to protect us.

Firstly, and most importantly, the EU, the FDA, and most Western governments require manufacturers to use safe substances in their processes. This is covered by the use of the term "FOOD GRADE PLASTIC." Basically, anything designed for use with food has strict rules around it. This is true of clingfilm (shrinkwrap), too.

If you are not sure whether one of your containers is made of food-grade plastic, and you want to store your bean sprouts in it (I'm assuming you're definitely going to grow some) have a look on the packaging. Safe plastic symbols are stamped in a triangle of arrows. The food grade plastic are 1, 2, 4, or 5.

This is correct at time of going to press, but if you want to keep up to date, there are a number of websites that give detailed advice on this, including *www.wrap.org.uk/* and Wikkihow.com.

There is also a huge debate going on at present about one specific chemical, Bisphenol A, or BPA, as it is popularly known. It's used to make things like refillable drinks bottles and food storage containers as well as protective coatings and linings for cans.

France has banned BPA from food packaging, citing health fears as the reason. Canada has put bisphenol A on its list of toxic substances, while the US Environmental Protection Agency (EPA) has marked it as a "chemical of concern." However, in January 2015, the EU published a report that concluded BPA poses no health risk to consumers of any age group, including unborn children, infants, and adolescents, at current exposure levels (although it did reduce the safe level of BPA to 4 μg/kg of bw/day).

The problem for many of us is that we have no idea what that means in practice. Can I have one can of beans and a swig of water from a water bottle a day? One odd source of BPA was the thermal paper from till receipts, so from now on they can keep them!

This debate is so hot that companies that do take BPA out of their products are advertising the fact as an obvious selling point. The new worry is that they will replace the BPA with other chemicals that are just as bad. So at the time of writing, the best option is to go for food-grade plastic, as this is constantly monitored. To be honest, I'm broken-hearted about this, as I love my tinned coconut milk and sardines. Some companies have begun to use BPA-free tins, but typically, the products are very expensive!

Synthetic Estrogen in Cleaning Products

Most cleaning products are often unashamedly full of chemicals that kill natural substances. Many have big warnings on the side saying that if you accidentally swallow some you must rush to hospital, while others suggest that you shouldn't even inhale them. Yet we splash them around our homes, pleased at how clean we are. My bottle of bleach has a big "DANGER" sign on the label, whilst my sink unblocker just goes for the skull and cross bones.

Nobody wants to give up bleach completely, but there are compromises you can make and still be clean. Firstly, there are a number of non-toxic cleaning products on the market, including Bio D, Ecover, and Method. In the UK, the supermarket Waitrose now offers a whole range of ecological cleaning products. And yes, before you ask, they *are* more expensive, but not to the planet or our health. In the US it's even better, with a large range of non-toxic cleaning products widely available at different price points in supermarkets and health food stores.

Secondly, many natural substances, such as lemon, (very acidic, great for cutting through grease), vinegar (wonderful for cleaning windows), and bicarbonate of soda (gets stains out of clothes) can substitute for cleaning products. A number of websites and books cover this subject. Look it up. You'll be amazed.

Natural Ways to Rid Ourselves of Toxins

I know we think of toxins as a modern phenomenon, but they are not; they have always been in the environment, we have always eaten things that might be bad for us, and we have often accidentally poisoned ourselves. Luckily, the body has ways to neutralize, eliminate, and rebalance.

When scientist Katherine Milton looked at wild monkey diets, she found the plants the monkeys were eating contained lots of natural toxins, but the sheer amount of good plants they ingested were washing the bad stuff out of their bodies. [261, 262]

This proves that we evolved with natural mechanisms to help us get rid of hazardous substances. Sadly, we are no longer able to munch through piles of green leaves every day, the way our monkey ancestors did. Milton says that, even if we wanted to, we literally don't have the stomach for it anymore, as our digestive systems evolved to receive smaller amounts of nutrient-dense, easy-to-digest, often cooked food.

Clearly, to get the best of both worlds, what we need is something that contains high amounts of these natural plant chemicals, which you only have to eat a small amount of in order to get massive benefits and which is easily digestible. Well, that's what sprouted greens and beans are!

We have already seen that brassica sprouts help the body excrete more airborne pollutants.[98] Another study took two groups of young smokers and gave half of them a diet rich in kaempferol and quercetin (found in brassica sprouts[92]). After just six days, the group that ate a diet rich in kaempferol and quercetin had less DNA damage, and the study concluded that a diet rich in polyphenols (a posh word for lovely plant compounds) could "decrease the risk of chronic diseases by reducing oxidative stress."[263]

Obviously, we must all limit our exposure to chemicals as much as possible, but to ensure we get rid of those toxins we can't avoid, we must eat as many plant compounds as possible. All sprouts are known for their antioxidant effect, but brassica sprouts have particular compounds that help us clear them out. So grow radish, broccoli, or cress.

Fasting is an ancient way of clearing the body, which modern science is now proving to be an invaluable tool.[264, 265] So if you are seriously worried about your toxin levels, it's another natural thing you can try. Certain health conditions make fasting unsuitable; check with your doctor first.

CHAPTER 18

Hormone-Rich Recipes and Dining Suggestions

So far in this book, I have talked about plant estrogen and progesterone, cancer-fighting compounds such as glucosinolates, and plant nutrients that wash toxins out of our body.

We want them all, right?

This chapter will show you how to make easy adjustments to your diet to get the maximum amount of wonderful foods containing all these qualities with the minimum of effort. I have included old-fashioned recipes, so you can see just how big a part of our culinary heritage peas, beans, and lentils are. My mother told me she always ate lentils as a child, but by the time I came along they were considered the preserve of vegetarians. These recipes prove that we can have both.

Menopause Porridge

- Oats soaked overnight
- Linseeds (flaxseeds) – sprouted or soaked, if possible
- Pumpkin seeds
- Sunflower seeds
- Milk or water
- Dried apricots or dates to sweeten

There's nothing like an overnight hot flush to make you want to start your day with menopause porridge. There are several different versions, depending on how much you can think ahead. You could make your traditional porridge and add flaxseeds that have been sprouted for just a few days to the mix. If you haven't got sprouted flaxseeds ready, just grind up them up dry and stir in a tablespoonful; you'll hardly notice. If you have pumpkin or sunflower seeds, add them, too. Either grind them, or make sure you chew them, otherwise they will go straight through you.

Even better is to soak oats and seeds overnight, then cook them on the hob in the morning. They won't take as long to cook and will be even more digestible and better for you.

Used chopped apricots or dates to sweeten. These are both rich in progesteronic compounds, so they are a lovely complement to the rest of the porridge. You can also make an apricot or date paste to add, like jam but with none of the sugar. Do this by blending dried fruit with a little water. That's it. Wonderful.

MENOPAUSE MUESLI

- Rolled grains (buckwheat, oats, or rye)
- Your favourite dried fruits (apricots and dates are best)
- Nuts and seeds
- Soaked chia seeds – optional
- Fresh seasonal fruit as a topper

I know it's easy to buy muesli in the shops, and please do that if you have no time. But making your own is so much cheaper, and you can customize it to your exact liking. If you like it very sweet, add more fruit; for a very earnest muesli, add more grains and simple seeds; for a luxurious breakfast experience, add more nuts and even some honey.

The big trick to making muesli more digestible is to soak it overnight, either in plain water or your favourite milk, or do as I do and soak the muesli in a mixture consisting of one tablespoonful of natural yoghurt combined with water; the grains and seeds start to predigest, the yoghurt starts to ferment, and all in all, you wake up to an interesting brew in your breakfast bowl.

Maximilian Bircher-Benne who invented muesli as part of his cancer fighting diet *always* soaked everything overnight. This has somehow been forgotten.

SPROUT SALT

- Red clover or alfalfa
- Broccoli, cress, or radish
- Fenugreek

- Mineral salt
- Dried seaweed

This is a lovely hormonal sprinkle to put on your food. Gather as many different green sprouts as you can. Include some spicy ones, such as cress and radish (or both), and add some ancient menopause healers, such as red clover or alfalfa, which will calm the spiciness down. Even add some fenugreek, if you want to give your libido a boost.

It's very simple to do. You clean off most of the hulls, then you dehydrate your sprouts. If you don't own a dehydrator, put them in the lowest oven setting that you can until they are completely dried out. It doesn't take long.

To make sprout salt, you need to add a tablespoon of mineral salt and some dried seaweed (although some people think seaweed alone is salty enough). Grind it all up together, and put it in an airtight container. Take it on holiday and anywhere you can't get access to your normal sprouts. Sprinkle it on food. No one will know you are taking your HRT right in front of them.

SPROUT-VEGETABLE COMBINATIONS

- Broccoli with spicy sprouts
- Carrots with red clover sprouts
- Cauliflower with cress sprouts
- Green beans with red sango radish sprouts

Just when you thought vegetables couldn't be any better for you, try adding sprouts to them; it turns normal vegetable dishes into a superfood surprise.

Just a handful of green sprouts lounging decorously over steamed vegetables gives a healthy yet luxurious-looking meal.

Try steamed broccoli with added broccoli sprouts for that intense broccoli experience. Cauliflower draped in cress sprouts turns it into an exotic delight. For a striking colour contrast, try deep red sango radish sprouts on any green vegetables.

The reason to mix brassica vegetables with spicy sprouts is that it will mean more of the cancer-fighting compounds in the vegetables will be converted to their active form. We saw in Chapter 16 that myrosinase is destroyed by cooking, so the spicy sprouts will step in and make up the difference.

Scientists keen to find ways to maximize the cancer-fighting potential of vegetables have tested this and suggest that we eat broccoli with mustard powder[266] or mustard seeds,[267] but sprouts are a much more glamorous way to achieve this. This might be why spicy sprouts, such as cress, radish, or broccoli, have traditionally been used for garnish, as they add a zing to any meal.

We don't have to stop there, though. Carrots dressed with red clover are a cheeky mix, and alfalfa makes a fine garnish on any food. Try different combinations to give your taste buds a treat.

BRASSICA AND MUNG BEAN HORMONE-RICH STIR-FRY

Stir-fries are a wonderfully healthy and delicious way to eat brassica vegetables, such as broccoli, cauliflower, or cabbage, into a kaempferol-rich delight.

Chop vegetables very thinly, along with onions, leeks, or garlic (which are prebiotic and will help fermentation). Heat pan with a good fat or oil until it sizzles, and add the above with any other vegetables you like. Carrots go very nicely, and courgettes and peppers are lovely. All will add different vitamins and healthy plant compounds.

If you like meat, thinly slice a small amount. If not, use big, meaty mushrooms. Right at the last minute, add your mung beans and season to taste. Serve with rice.

If you like a more juicy stir-fry, pour in some water, add some bouillon, and let it bubble for a while to allow the flavours to sink in. Thicken with arrowroot powder if desired, then sprinkle sprouts on top and serve.

HOW TO USE SPROUTED BEANS IN PLACE
OF DRIED BEANS IN RECIPES

Bean stews, Mexican bean dishes, haricot bean bake, bean burgers—lots of recipes using dry beans require you to cook them by boiling them. Sadly, you can't simply substitute sprouted beans without losing some of the texture of the original dish. There is a compromise, though: soaking and sprouting for just one day gives you a bit of both. Beans will still be "beany" but will be better for you.

Just soaking beans overnight will help. When you do, notice how rank the water gets. That's the beans sloughing off any anti-nutrients. They are already changing and growing. So get out your favourite bean recipes, and give it a go.

ADUKI BEAN BROWNIES

I've always liked the deep rich red of adukis, and it turns out they are the sweetest of all the beans, and slightly creamy too, so perfect for desserts of all kinds.

- 1 cup of aduki beans, soaked, sprouted for 1–3 days and lightly cooked
- ½ cup chopped dates (or ¾ of a cup if you have a sweet tooth)
- ¼ cup cocoa powder, macca powder, or shredded coconut
- 3 tbs olive oil, coconut oil, or melted butter
- 2 eggs

Sprout the aduki beans for as long as you can bear to wait. The longer you sprout them, the less dense the beans will be. In a food processor or blender combine the dates with the oil and eggs, and blend until they form a paste. Add the aduki beans and blend again until creamy, and *finally* add the cocoa powder, macca powder, or coconut.

Pour in the mixture into a greaseproof dish and bake for half an hour at 180C/350F. When they come out of the oven, let them cool for 10–15 minutes, then cut them into squares. You can double up this recipe and make lots of them and keep them in the fridge or freezer.

HAS-BEAN CAKE

I adapted this recipe from a basic banana cake and couldn't believe how perfectly it turned out. It is not only delicious but vegan, gluten free, and contains no added sugar, so *everyone* can enjoy it. I have been feeding it to friends and telling them it's called Has-Bean Cake, 'cos it has beans in it!' –otherwise you really might forget!

- 6 ripe bananas
- ¾ cup raisins or sultanas (add more if you like a really fruity cake or you can use chopped dates as an alternative)
- 1 cup aduki beans, sprouted for 1–3 days
- 1 cup oats

- 3 tbs olive oil, coconut oil or melted butter.
- Chopped nuts to sprinkle on top (optional)

Put the bananas and oil in a food processor using the S blade, and process until smooth. (You can do it in a blender, but you need to chop the bananas up quite small and possibly add extra oil to get it to turn over). Add in the oats and aduki beans, and continue blending. Switch off the blender and stir in the raisins or sultanas. Pour into a greaseproof dish, sprinkle on nuts, and bake until firm to the touch. Usually 30 minutes and 180C/350F.

Lovely Lentil Bread

This bread has no wheat or yeast, yet somehow remains very "bready" and satisfying. It's possible that you could make this recipe with any legume, but I think lentil is the most lovely.

- 1 cup lentils, sprouted 1–3 days. No need to cook first.
- 2 ½ tbs psyllium husk
- 4 eggs
- 1 tsp sea salt
- 1 tsp baking powder
- 1 tbs ground flaxseeds (soaked, if possible)

Separate egg yolks from the whites, and whisk the whites until fluffy in a blender or food processor (this aerates the bread beautifully). Add the yolks back in, then the sprouted lentils. Finally add the salt, baking powder, psyllium husks, and ground flaxseeds.

Note: the flaxseeds and psyllium husks are quite dense, so you might need to stir them in if you are using a blender and it won't turn over.

Pour the mixture into the prepared tin (either greased or lined with greaseproof paper), and bake for 40 minutes at 180C/ 350F.

This bread doesn't keep as well as normal bread, so I slice it up and keep it in the freezer. It defrosts very quickly when you need it, or you can pop it in the toaster.

Heavenly Hormonal Health Dip / Side Dish

- Red clover sprouts
- Capers

- Herb salt
- Sage
- Organic natural (plain) yoghurt

Mix all the ingredients into the natural yoghurt. Blend, if you like it smooth. It tastes fantastic. Everything in it will work together in your body to beat those hot flushes, prevent that cancer, and build those strong bones. For a tangier version, use broccoli or radish sprouts, or mix them together for a bit of everything.

PROGESTERONIC FLAPJACKS

Basically, these are normal flapjacks but with honey, apricots, and linseeds to give them a hormonal punch. Using honey instead of sugar is a lovely way to give yourself a healthy sweet treat.

- 1 cup butter
- ½ cup honey
- 3 cups oats
- Pinch of salt
- ½ cup linseeds
- ¾ cup dried apricots or dates roughly chopped

Melt the honey and butter together in a pan over a gentle heat. Then turn the heat off, and stir in the oats, sunflower seeds, and apricots, mixing with a wooden spoon so that all the ingredients are well combined. Pour the mixture into the prepared tin (either greased or lined with greaseproof paper). Bake in the preheated oven 180C/ 350F/ for 25 minutes, or until golden brown. Remove from the tin and cut into squares when completely cool.

CHICKPEA HUMMUS

- 1 cup soaked chickpeas or 1 ½ cups sprouted chickpeas
- 2 tbs tahini
- 2 tbsp extra virgin olive oil
- 2 large cloves garlic
- Juice of 2 medium lemons
- 2 tsp paprika (for garnish)
- Salt to taste

I always think that making a big bowl of hummus and serving it to friends is a joyous way to live, so much better than the tiny little pots you can buy, which might be processed. There are so many variations, too.

Some people do this recipe completely raw; others prefer to cook their chickpeas. If cooking, boil chickpeas for at least an hour, until they are soft (soaked and sprouted chickpeas take much less time than their dried counterparts). If raw, sprout the chickpeas until they have a 1cm root (but no longer as they become bitter).

Put all the ingredients in a blender and whizz them up until they are smooth. If it is too thick, add a little water. Sprinkle on paprika. For a smoother hummus, remove chickpea husks first. Enjoy.

FLAVONOID-FULL GREEN SMOOTHIE

- Any green vegetables (celery, cucumber, lettuce, kale, spinach)
- Any sprouted greens (flax, red clover, broccoli, cress)
- Dandelions, nettles (young, if in season, or new growth)
- Any fruit
- Natural yoghurt or sauerkraut

As mentioned above, until recently we ate an enormous range of foods, simply because we ate anything that was edible. A way to mimic this (and get all those weird and wonderful but not necessarily tasty things into your diet) is to have a green smoothie once a day.

If you use a combination of vegetables, sprouted greens (it's a great way to use them up if you have a glut), and wild greens from the garden, you will get a broad range of interesting plant nutrients and all important flavonoids.

Use whatever you have to hand—sprouts, vegetables, and wild foods.

Throw it all in the blender or smoothie maker, and blend until smooth.

If you don't have any natural yoghurt, try adding sauerkraut to help activate your gut bacteria. The fruit is there to make it taste better. Glug it down, and enjoy the rest of your day, knowing you have given your body what it needs.

Old-Fashioned Recipes

Lentils and Hock

- 2 cups brown lentils (soaked overnight, sprouted one day)
- 2 tbs olive oil
- 2 small diced onions
- 3 sticks celery sliced
- 3 carrots
- 3 cloves garlic chopped
- Salt and pepper
- 2 tbs chopped garlic
- Bay leaves, thyme and parsley
- 3 to 4 smoked ham hocks
- 1 litre chicken or vegetable stock

This is an old-fashioned recipe that has a bit of everything. Lentils for plant estrogen; garlic, parsley, and other herbs for plant progesterone; and vegetables for prebiotics.

Fry the onions, celery, garlic, and carrots over low heat until the onions are golden. Add the ham hocks and stock, and sprinkle on bay leaves and thyme. Cover and simmer for 1 hour.

Drain lentils and add them to the pan. Cook another 30 minutes. Take out the ham hocks and remove the meat from the bone, then add them back into the soup. Season with salt and pepper. Use the parsley as a garnish. Very yummy.

Pease Pudding
(also known as Pottage or Geordie Hummus!)

A very comforting old British dish that goes perfectly with salty gammon or is just as a lovely dip. It even has its own nursery rhyme to go with it:

Pease pudding hot,
Pease pudding cold,
Pease pudding in the pot, nine days old.
Some like it hot,
Some like it cold,

Some like it in the pot,
Nine days old.

There are various recipes. I prefer this one.

- 3 cups yellow split peas soaked overnight
- 1 onion
- Fresh herbs
- ½ cup butter
- 1 large egg
- Salt and freshly ground black pepper to taste (or vegetable bouillon)
- Vinegar or wine to taste

Soak the split peas in fresh water for 24 hours. Rinse and drain. Put in a pan with all the other ingredients apart from the vinegar. Simmer for 2 ½ hours. Don't let it boil dry. Drain the cooked split peas. Blend in a food processor, or press through a sieve or a potato ricer. Beat in the egg and butter, and season well. When you make it, you'll immediately understand its nickname, as it looks and tastes similar to hummus but somehow lacks the trendiness of the Mediterranean diet. We can change that!

OLD-FASHIONED LENTIL SOUP

- 6 cups chicken or vegetable stock
- 1 cup dried lentils (soaked overnight, then sprouted for one day)
- 2 tbs extra virgin olive oil
- 2 cloves fresh garlic, chopped
- 3 celery stalks, chopped
- 2 large onions chopped
- 3 large carrots, chopped
- 1 tube tomato puree
- Salt and pepper, to taste
- Parsley for garnish

Fry all the vegetables in the oil until soft. Add the stock, tomato puree, and lentils, and simmer for an hour. Garnish with parsley. Serve with Lentil Bread (see recipe above). Blending is optional.

Pea and Ham Soup

I think a lot of people went off this soup because the tinned variety was truly awful. However, freshly cooked, it's an absolute delight.

There are two versions you can make: a slow, luxurious, old-fashioned (and very economical version) and a quick one for when in a hurry.

Slow Version

- 3 cups dried marrowfat peas
- 1.5–2kg fresh ham (you can use the cheaper cuts for this)
- 4 carrots, peeled and chopped
- 2 large onions, peeled and chopped
- A few sprigs of fresh thyme
- Salt and pepper to taste (or bouillon)
- Fresh finely chopped parsley

Soak the marrowfat peas overnight, then boil them for an hour, and drain. Put the onions, vegetables, and bouillon in a pan with the ham and boil for two hours. Remove the ham shank and once cooled, take all the meat and fat off the bone, and cut into 2cm pieces before putting them back in the soup.

Add the marrowfat peas, and liquidize half of it. Stir the liquidized portion into the remaining soup for a nice, thick, chunky texture. Add the rest of the marrow fat peas, and simmer for 30 minutes.

Some recipes say you should leave it in the fridge overnight to enhance the flavour. Some say you should add potatoes to the pot. Some say you should thicken with arrowroot. Basically, you can do what you like with it, and it will still be delicious.

Quick Version

- Ready-cooked ham off the bone, cut into small slices
- Packet of frozen peas
- 2 potatoes, chopped small
- 2 carrots, chopped
- 2 onions, chopped
- Knob of butter
- Vegetable bouillon
- ½ litre of water

Fry the onions in the butter, and when golden brown, add the potato and stir until the potatoes are all coated in butter. Add water and bouillon. Simmer until softened.

Add frozen peas, and bring back to the boil. Allow to simmer for another 5 minutes. Remove from the heat, and blend until smooth. Stir in the ham and serve.

SAUSAGE AND BEAN STEW

- Cup of haricot beans (soaked overnight and sprouted for one day)
- 1 tbs olive oil
- 8 pork sausages
- 1 onion, chopped
- 3 garlic cloves, crushed
- 1 sprig rosemary leaves, chopped
- Jar of tomato puree
- 2 cups chicken stock
- Large bunch of spinach
- Parsley, chopped
- Salt and black pepper

Prick sausages, and fry with the onion on low heat, turning frequently until onions are golden and sausages are brown (about 15 minutes).

Add tomato and garlic, and stir until simmering. Pour in the chicken stock and simmer with the lid on.

At the last minute, wash and chop the spinach, lay it on the top of the stew, and let the steam cook it. Serve with parsley garnish.

Interesting variations include the addition of any root vegetables in season or different beans, such as chickpeas or aduki; the red of aduki beans against the green of the spinach looks lovely.

Having said all that, I knew someone who used to fry sausages and onions, and pour in a can of baked beans and a bit of stock and be done with it (and yes, it was delicious).

MENOPAUSE CHRISTMAS DINNER
(THAT YOU CAN HAVE EVERY WEEK, IF YOU LIKE)

Christmas dinner is great because you eat Brussels sprouts, (you could steam a few broccoli sprouts on top of them), sage and onion stuffing is wonderful (try adding lentil sprouts to them to make it even better for you), and lots of seasonal vegetables. For afters, have an old-fashioned plum pudding, rich in prunes, apricots, and spices, and probiotic natural yoghurt to convert it all to plant hormones. Or try having a nut and seed roast alternative for even more lovely nutrients.

EGGSHELL MINERAL MIX

I took expensive mineral supplements for years until I found out that you can grind up eggshells and take half a teaspoon a day for a marvellous mineral mix. It's particularly full of calcium, and tests have shown it has positive effects on bone and cartilage, prevention of osteoporosis, [268] and demineralizing teeth. [269]

All the way through this book, I have been talking about our ability to absorb nutrients, and these tested as "similar or better than vitamin pills." [270] This information is so exciting, some Japanese scientists have suggested that we should fortify all of our foods with them. [271]

To make this mineral mix, you need to save a few organic egg shells (hopefully, you can afford to use organic, as they are saving you money on vitamin pills). Wash them and then put them in the oven at 300 degrees for 25 minutes. Some websites say you need to boil them, too, but I can't see that it adds anything. Pulverize them up in a grinder (coffee grinders work), and keep them in an airtight jar. Half a teaspoonful of eggshell mix a day provides the following minerals:

- Calcium   900mg
- Magnesium   24.mg
- Phosphorus   8.4mg
- Potassium   8.0mg
- Sodium   9.0mg

As you can see, it's not just about calcium. It will help with our magnesium levels, too, which is good because we need both (and it will help us utilize vitamin D). I have a friend who mixes hers with honey to help it go down, I just swallow mine with water.

HOW TO SNEAK MORE PLANT ESTROGEN AND PLANT PROGESTERONE INTO YOUR DIET

If the recipes above seem too complicated, here are some simple ways to raise your plant hormone levels.

Garlic is a great estrogenic food to add to your diet, I try to have a clove of raw garlic a day—that's right, I don't have a boyfriend at the moment! You can also eat garlic bread, or add garlic to dressings.

The way to get more isoflavones into your diet is to eat more legumes, such as beans and peas and lentils. We have a long tradition in Britain of eating garden peas and mushy peas with everything, and we can bring that back. Most health stores sell tins of ready cooked organic beans, organic hummus, bean burgers, and other bean dips. While you're in there, look out for tins of sugar-free baked beans, and enjoy them on toast.

If you want more coumestrol in your diet, (which don't forget is the plant estrogen that's 30 times stronger than isoflavones), try and get into bean sprout dishes. This is a wonderful excuse to have a takeaway from your local Chinese restaurant. Some people don't like the MSG so, of course, you can grow your own mung beans to a longer length to put in stir fries or to make a chow mein.

Always include at least one brassica vegetable with your meal for the cancer fighting compounds. If you're eating out, most restaurants serve broccoli (it's very fashionable). When you are at home, always add a garnish to your meal. Alfalfa and red clover are rich sources of all of the plant estrogens, as noted earlier.

If you are particularly looking for plant progesterone, capers top the list of kaempferol-containing foods. Best known as a pizza and pasta ingredient, capers are rather nice in salads as they are very tangy little beans. Incredibly, they contain 135.56 mg of kaempferol per 100g, so try munching through a jar of capers a month.

Meanwhile, the biggest source of apigenin is parsley. Parsley was traditionally added as a garnish to many dishes. It's another thing that's been forgotten and is so easy to bring back. Mixing parsley with garlic minimizes the smell of the garlic too.[272]

If you struggle to remember to eat your sprouts then get into mixing your sprouted greens with normal food. How about having egg and cress sandwiches, salmon and cress sandwiches, anything and cress? It adds a spiciness and wonderful plant hormones to everything you eat.

If you like condiments such as mustard, rather than go for the commercially prepared kind, why not grind up some mustard seeds, or better still get some mustard greens, which are rich in lignans and kaempferol. Horseradish is also very high in kaempferol, so horseradish sauce is a must if you can take the heat!

Western food doesn't have to be bland. Open up that baguette, pop in some mung and lentil sprouts, close it again, and you'll hardly know they are there. Add a sprouted garnish to your pizza, and make sure you always have capers on it—you might even like them.

Avocados are a wonderful food, too, as they are rich in plant hormones. Have them mashed on toast, add them to your salad, or have them on their own with a little cider vinegar, a few sprouts, and some garlic. Mmm... lovely.

If you don't want sprouts with your main meal, how about making a salad starter? Or crudities and a dip? You'll feel very posh. If you can't be bothered with that, just eat a handful of sprouts before you eat your evening meal. You'll feel like you have earned whatever you are eating, and enjoy it even more.

I'm not saying that this will cure all your ills, but it's a start, and if it makes even a bit of difference to your health and hot flushes, you might be encouraged to look at what else you can change.

Do what you can today. Don't worry what you can or can't do tomorrow. Add some sprouts to your life in any way that you can.

PART FOUR
– PRACTICAL –

CHAPTER 19

WHAT IS SPROUTING? HOW DO I DO IT?

Finally we get to the bit where you learn how to sprout! One question I get asked a lot is: What's the difference between a bean sprout and a baby green? Beans sprouts are beans that you water for just a few days until a root forms and they're ready to eat. Sprouted baby greens, often called salad greens, are grown until they have a root, a green shoot, and a little double leaf. They take longer, usually 5–7 days, and can be used like lettuce.

WHY SPROUT?

Obviously I have been banging on about why you should sprout throughout this book, but for anyone who has turned to this section first, here is an overview.

Humans have been growing sprouts for thousands of years, using them as both food and medicine. NASA has even experimented with growing sprouts in space. Why not? Sprouts and baby greens are quick and easy to grow. They need no soil or compost, yet manage to have ounce per ounce more vitamins and minerals than their full grown counterparts. [273, 114] Great for astronauts and earth dwellers alike.

Sprouts are a local food. There are lots of superfoods around at the moment, but they all seem to come from Peru or the Amazon rainforest. Bean sprouts and baby greens are superfoods that you can grow yourself, all year round, in your house, with minimal effort, at a fraction of the cost.

Sprouts are living food. Most people eat them raw. Even when you store them in the fridge for a week, they still keep growing, very slowly. They just think it is a cold spell and can't wait to be warmed up. That means that they can still pass their living plant enzymes on to you.

Sprouts are so nutritious because when you water a bean or seed, nutrients intended to feed the baby plant are broken down into the simplest form of proteins, vitamins, enzymes, minerals, and trace elements. [274] This is called "predigestion. [114]

Normally, when you cook dry beans and pulses, you have to boil them vigorously to start with. This is because they contain toxins that upset our digestive systems. These are called "anti-nutrients." Sadly, cooking doesn't get rid of them all, which is why beans make you fart. More seriously, they reduce our absorption of minerals and trace elements, including iron, zinc, calcium, and manganese.[275, 276, 277] With most sprouts (apart from some of the bigger beans, such as chickpeas), this neutralization process happens automatically and naturally during the growing process. As the plants spring into life, toxins are sloughed off and anti-nutrients are discarded.

This all means that grown on your window ledge, your beans and baby greens are the freshest, most healthy foods you can ever eat.

Don't forget that sprouts grow so fast that children find them fascinating. It's a great way to get young people interested in growing and eating natural food.

WHAT CAN I GROW SPROUTS IN?

THE NO-SPEND OPTION: If you want to try sprouting without spending any money, it's easy to grow them in sieves, bowls, jars, and tubs. Usually, anything from the kitchen is good because it will be made of food-grade plastic. That means that it doesn't contain nasty chemicals that can leak onto your sprouts. Beans sprout in almost anything. Because you only sprout them until they have a root, they don't need any light and can be tightly packed in. Baby greens want light so they can green up and find something their roots can attach to, so they can stand up.

Household sieves (plastic not metal) and old vegetable steamers are particularly good because greens can root through the holes. This is the way we always sprouted before specialist equipment was invented. I certainly started off growing sprouts in random things about the house, and so can you. Have a poke round your cupboards and see what you can find.

FOOD GRADE PAPER: You probably grew sprouted mustard and cress on blotting paper as a kid, and you can do a modern version of that today by buying food grade paper. Normal paper contains bleaches and dyes that can leak onto your sprouts, so food grade is a must. Cress, in particular, loves to be grown on paper because the seeds are sticky and the paper is perfect for them to stick to. This also makes them easy to water without them being washed away.

Food-grade paper that has been passed fit for use with food will have the knife and fork symbol on the packet. The great thing about sprouting on paper is that sprouts need much less watering. You just have to wet the paper every time it dries out. This is usually more at first, as the seeds suck up the paper, but less as time goes on. You can double up sheets of paper, and that will cut down on watering.

This method of sprouting is perhaps the simplest, plus they are also easy to take on holiday. It's so light to carry a couple of sheets of paper and a few seeds and stick them on a plate in your caravan or hotel room (that will surprise the chambermaid!)

TRAYS: Specialist sprouting trays are available from most health food shops and can be bought both new and second-hand online. They come in various sizes and are sold in stacks of two or three slatted trays (the slats are so that water can flow through) and a drip tray underneath to catch it. Some provide a lid but unless it's transparent, it can stop your baby greens from getting light.

I use an old clear plastic tray as a lid as it keeps the air flowing and lets the light in. In-between each growth cycle, you need to wash trays in very hot water and scrub the slats to make sure they are clear of debris.

Trays theoretically last forever, but they do suffer wear and tear and can eventually crack. So you will need to buy new ones every few years. If you have a dishwasher and want to use it to wash your sprouting trays, make sure you only buy those described as "dishwasher safe." Trays are great for saving space as they stack. You can have your mung and lentil on the lower levels and your green sprouts at the top. You can also line trays with food grade paper to cut down on watering. Trays will need watering at least twice daily, and you have to tip trays to the side to make sure they are well drained, otherwise the seeds can clog the slats and get waterlogged, causing mould.

BAGS: Sprouting bags are usually made from organic hemp (which is naturally antifungal), flax, cotton, or nylon (which is easy to clean). They come with a string, so you can hang them over your bath or sink. To water your sprouts, you simply dunk the bag in a bowl of water twice a day, or run it under the tap.

Bags are a great way to grow any bean sprouts. They are portable, clean, and easy to care for. Bags last a long time and can be washed in the washing machine at high temperatures. Bags are also easy to travel with. You can hang them on the handles of your bike or keep them outside your tent when you're camping. I put mine in a plastic bag in my suitcase when I go away and unpack them the moment I get there.

You can't grow greens in bags because of the lack of light or ability to root. But for a plentiful supply of beans, bags are perfect.

SPECIALIST SPROUTING JARS: Specialist sprouting jars are available from health food outlets and online. They look like a normal jam jar but have a special top and base to keep them at the right angle to enable drainage. Pop your beans in to soak, drain, and water twice a day. Non-specialist sprouting jars are basically any jar you can find. Jars are portable and take up little space, but most people only use them for growing beans, as baby greens prefer more air and growing space. Also sprouts can get a bit sweaty in jars, whereas bags and trays allow air to circulate.

TUBS: Tubs are great for growing in bulk. They are especially suited for growing beans. You can grow some greens, such as alfalfa, but they do not green up as much as those grown in trays, and they need to be kept cool or watered frequently. Basically, the hotter the tubs get, the more watering your sprouts will need.

I'll just say again: you need to make sure it is food grade plastic (non–food grade plastic could have quite harmful chemicals, which is why they differentiate). So no growing in old buckets or cat litter trays (as someone once proudly told me they were doing). If you need to grow in bulk, this is the best method. Make sure they are clear plastic, to give them a chance. This is a bit like "factory farming"; it will do the job, but the sprouts won't be as happy!

AUTOMATIC SPROUTERS: For people who don't have the time to water their sprouts, automatic sprouters are a wonderful thing. You fill them with water, plug them in, and they will sprinkle your sprouts every few hours. You can grow anything you like in them. I have yet to find a sprout that won't grow in an automatic sprouter (but I haven't tried cress which probably prefers paper).

There are a few on the market. With most of them, you will need to change the water once a day, as it is recycled round after each watering, so it just gets more and more rank as time goes by.

This is especially true in the first stage of growing seeds, as the sprouts are sloughing off all the growth inhibitors and toxins naturally present. Later in the sprouting process, you can get away with longer. Automatic sprouters can be expensive to buy (although you can get them second-hand), and they use electricity and make a noise when they are watering. You also have to keep them in a place that is near water, electricity, and light. The kitchen is obviously ideal for most people, although many modern flats have kitchens without windows, which makes it a problem.

WHERE DO I BUY BEANS AND SEEDS FROM?

Red clover, broccoli, cress and fenugreek are rarely available on the high street, so it's best to get them from specialist sprouting websites (see resources). You can get them from eBay, but if you do, make sure they are organic and meant for sprouting, rather than for gardening, as they are not subject to the rigorous testing that seeds meant for sprouting are. Both the EU and FDA have rules and guidance for seed suppliers.

Sprouting seeds tend to come in 100g or 500g packets. The amount of seeds you need to sprinkle on the bottom of a 6-inch tray is 8–10g, depending on how thick you like them. So as you can see, 500g will give you 50 trays of sprouts. Seeds can be delicate, so I keep my large packets in the fridge and make sure the packet is sealed.

You can get aduki, mung bean, lentils, flaxseeds, and alfalfa seeds from the whole food store. I buy them organic—again because I mainly eat them raw. Beans are bigger and cheaper, but you use them up more quickly.

HARVESTING YOUR SPROUTS AND WASHING THE SEEDS OFF

Later in this chapter I will go into detail about each individual sprout, but no matter what you grow, they can all be kept in the fridge once they are ready. They usually last for about a week, although studies have shown that broccoli sprouts refrigerated for two weeks still had half of their cancer-fighting content.[278]

With alfalfa and red clover, you will need to rinse off the husks before you eat them. The reason is that they contain trace amounts of arsenic (alfalfa) and L-canavanine (red clover). It's not as dramatic as it sounds, as it is

138

largely neutralized during the sprouting process. Even if you ate unsprouted seeds, you would have to eat them in massive amounts to have any bad effects, so you don't have to go crazy and make sure every husk is removed; rinsing them under the tap is enough.

If you want to be more careful, you can put your crop in a bowl of water, jiggle them about, and the seeds will rise to the top and you can pour them off. The thing to note is that the studies on the toxicity of seeds are done just on the seeds and not on the sprouts. So you might come across old books that say "Don't sprout alfalfa." What they mean is, don't sprout it for just a few days, like you do with beans, and eat the whole thing. Eating the green sprouted plant with the seeds washed off is not only fine but nutritious.

There is no need to wash the husks from beans such as mung, lentil, and aduki. They are very good for you (more about this later). Fenugreek seeds can be used whole (and are in Asian cookery), as can flaxseeds. So you can eat them at any stage of the sprouting process. I have never read about any problem with eating broccoli, mustard, or cress hulls, but I do rinse mine.

SHOULD I STACK TRAYS?

You can stack trays (grow sprouts on top of each other) for all the different beans. Fenugreek, alfalfa, linseed, and red clover can also be stacked, but as they all want to get to the light you could try rotating them. I find broccoli really only likes growing in the top tray, but you can grow more tolerant sprouts underneath. All of the beans and legumes happily grow underneath, as they don't need any light. If you buy a stack of three trays, you might as well fill them all up, as it doesn't take any extra time to water them.

CAN I JUST EAT THE SEEDS AND NOT SPROUT THEM?

Apart from fenugreek, linseed, and the beans, which can go straight in the cooking pot, the answer is NO. Even if you are cooking with any of them, it's much better if you soak them overnight first, as it starts the growing process, including shedding of toxins, which, as we have seen, increases the digestibility.

WHERE SHOULD I GROW THEM?

Always grow sprouts where you can see them, otherwise, believe me, you'll forget to water them. Baby greens need indirect light. Some people keep their sprouts in the bathroom and water them when they go to the loo—after washing their hands, of course. If the sprouts are in an out-of-the-way place, set the timer on your phone as a reminder to water them. Once you get into the cycle of growing, you will feel sad any week that you forget.

WATERING

I often get asked whether it's okay to use tap water, and what I reply is that you should use the best water you can. That might be tap water, and that's okay; it's better than not having sprouts. I tend to soak my sprouts in filtered water, because that's when they absorb the most water, then use tap water after that. We must all do what works for us.

Always water your green sprouts gently; if you pour water directly onto them, you might dislodge the roots. A way to get round this is to put an empty tray on top and allow the water to drip through it. I tip trays of sprouts and plates of cress to the side to make sure they drain.

Some people prefer to spray their sprouts. It's easy to keep a bottle of filtered water next to them. Spraying may take slightly longer, but it cuts down on having to drain them. Do make sure you get every sprout wet, and if you are spraying cress, that the paper gets soaked, too. Spraying is not suitable for sprouting bags. You need to either run them under the tap or dunk them in a bowl of water.

SHOULD I COOK SPROUTED GREENS AND BEANS?

In terms of digestibility, we have seen sprouting significantly cuts down on toxins, whilst increasing their vitamin, mineral, and antioxidant activity. Some people do find it hard to digest bigger beans such as chickpeas, and some writers, such as Steve Meyerowitz (AKA Sproutman), suggest you can cook them lightly. If you do cook them, sprouted beans need much less cooking than their unsprouted counterparts and are still much more nutritious.

As for baby greens, I have been eating them raw with no problem for years, but some people are worried about health scares (see more in FAQs). The good news is that you can steam them, as steaming leaves most of the nutrients intact. [279] In fact, there have been specific studies on cooking broccoli and its effect on the cancer-fighting glucosinolates. Microwaving and boiling came off worst; steaming was best, with stir-frying (without water) second.[280]

Plus as we have seen in the recipes section, you can drape red clover, broccoli, or cress sprouts over steaming cauliflower or broccoli. It really makes it look lovely as well as upping the nutritional content enormously. If you have a dinner party serve them up and *everyone* will be talking about it.

CHAPTER 20

How to Grow Mung, Lentil, Aduki, and Chickpea Sprouts

Basic Instructions

Soak beans, peas or lentils for at least 8–16 hours. After that, the water will start to fizz on top, which tells you they are not happy. The beans will almost double in size just from soaking, then quadruple during the sprouting process. Note: You can grow mung beans, lentils, and chickpeas together, but aduki beans take a little longer, so grow them separately.

Drain and put the beans into your sprouting bag, tray, jar, or tub.

Rinse them twice a day. Make sure they are well drained. Tip trays onto their sides. I dunk my sprouting bags under the tap.

A tiny root should start to grow within one day (it takes longer when it's cold). Watch these roots, and when they are as long as the bean itself, they are ready to be harvested (usually 2–3 days). Give them a final water and pop them in the fridge. They should keep for a week.

You can keep growing mung beans, and they will miraculously turn into Chinese-style bean sprouts. This is a great home-grown vegetable in its own right. To grow them, you just need to keep on watering them for up to 12 days.

If you are going to do this, you need to keep them in the dark or they will start to grow a green shoot, and we really only want the root. So just tie up your sprouting bag, or put a dark lid on your tub (prick holes in it so they can breathe).

Put weights on them if you want them to be straighter—that's how the Chinese do it. Some companies also use ethane gas to fatten them up, but there's nothing wrong with a thinner, curly sprout; they are wonderful either raw or in a stir fry. Feed them to friends who will be so impressed you grew them yourself.

WHICH VITAMINS, MINERALS, AND PLANT HORMONES DO THEY CONTAIN?

All beans, peas, and lentils contain high amounts of all the different plant estrogens, especially isoflavones. This is particularly true of sprouted chickpeas,[281] which contains at least seven different forms of isoflavones,[282, 283] while mung beans are one of the richest sources of coumestrol. All beans have slightly different qualities, so it's worth varying them. There has been more research into mung beans, so the others might be just as good but less researched.

Mung beans contain 20 percent protein, calcium, iron, magnesium, phosphorus, potassium, vitamins A, C, and E, riboflavin, and niacin.

Chickpeas have 20 percent protein, vitamins A, C, and E, iron, calcium, and magnesium.

Lentils have 25 percent protein, vitamins A, B, C, and E, iron, calcium, and phosphorus.

Aduki beans have 25 percent protein, all of the amino acids (except for tryptophan), vitamin A, C, and E, iron, niacin, and calcium.

OTHER REASONS TO GROW MUNG, LENTIL, AND ADUKI BEANS OR CHICKPEAS

We have already seen that beans are great for the heart and are filled with antioxidants.[284] Sprouted beans have such a lovely array of nutrients that the cosmetic industry is even using them in their skin preparations.[285]

A recent study showed that, in mung beans, vitamin C peaks on day 8, with up to 285 mg/100 g, which is almost 24 times higher than the initial concentration. However, their general antioxidant ability peaks on days 2–3,[286] so whenever you eat them they will be great for you, especially as all other nutrients are increased, too.[287] Added to this, sprouted mung beans have anti-tumour effects in mice,[288] along with anti-diabetic activity.[289]

Sprouted lentils give mung beans a run for their money. If you sprout them rather than cook them from their dry form, it increases their vitamin C content by 1,000 percent. Three-day-old lentil sprouts have 16.5mg vitamin C per 100g, and sprouting increases their antioxidant[290] and polyphenol content.[291] Just to remind you, polyphenols are a posh word for compounds that help protect us from bacteria and viruses, and that's protection we all could use.[292]

Aduki (also known as adzuki) beans are another ancient bean we've been eating since before records began. We have already seen that it is particularly associated with heart health, as it not only has lots of fibre but also helps lower blood pressure.[293] In mice, it has been shown to help reduce the symptoms of type 2 diabetes.[294] Aduki beans are a very attractive deep red colour. They are sweeter than other beans, so you can even make desserts with them (see recipe section). If you fancy a change, do give them a go.

Chickpeas are one of the oldest cultivated crops on the planet. They contain high-quality protein and several essential minerals.[295] Chickpeas have a distinctive taste that combines well in savoury dishes, not least in hummus, but do try chickpea curry or stew, too.

SHOULD I WASH THE HULLS OFF?

I used to tell people that the hulls and husks of beans and lentils were harmless fibre, but now I know that they are actually rather good for you.

One study found that mung bean hulls are an antioxidant in their own right.[117] Lentil fibre is great for the functioning of our digestion and also provides food for gut flora.[296] How great is it that they contain brilliant plant compounds and come with the right fibre to feed our gut bacteria? You don't get that in a supplement.

So, no, don't wash the hulls off, apart from if you are growing mung beans into a full Chinese-style sprout.

CHAPTER 21

How to Grow Alfalfa, Broccoli, Radish, and Red Clover Sprouts

Basic Instructions

I usually soak seeds overnight to give them a good start and let the seeds know that I mean business. They are small seeds and will double in size. You can get away with not soaking them as long as you water them thoroughly, but the tiny unsoaked seeds are much more likely to fall through the slats of the trays and cause wastage.

Drain and put them into your sprouting tray. I tend to have my green sprouts growing on the top of a stack of trays because they want the light, and have my beans growing underneath. If you find broccoli hard to grow, you could try not stacking at all and just have one layer. Broccoli are the most sensitive of all the sprouts but are very much worth the effort.

Keep the sprouting tray in a cool place (not on a radiator, for example) but not so cold that they won't grow.

Water and drain them 2–3 times a day. Experiment with different watering times and see what you can get away with—they sometimes need less in the winter. See the troubleshooting section below for more on this. If you don't water them enough, they will start to get a white mould on them. Always make sure you hold the tray to the side for a few seconds to allow all the water to drain, otherwise sprouts can drown.

If you grow seeds in a tray, the roots will burrow into the slats and the baby sprouts will stand up straight, reaching towards the light. If you grow them in a tub this can't happen, and they won't be as green.

Your crop will be ready in 5–8 days, depending upon the time of year. At the height of summer, you'll be amazed by how fast each batch is ready. Harvest them when they have a double leaf. Wash off most of the seed husks and put them into the fridge. They will keep for a week. If you feel kind, you could water them every few days, because they are all still alive in there, waiting for their moment!

WHICH VITAMINS, MINERALS, AND PLANT HORMONES DO THEY CONTAIN?

At the time of writing, red clover is known to be the richest source of all the different forms of isoflavones and of coumestrol, which is why supplement makers use it. As noted in Part One, it contains kaempferol, which guarantees you plant progesterone and other yet unidentified compounds that have progesteronic effects. Added to this, animal studies show that red clover is considered a "safe" estrogen, giving all its benefits without any of the dangers associated with too much estrogen.[83, 297]

Red clover contains 30 percent protein, vitamins A, B, C, and E, calcium, magnesium, potassium, iron, zinc, and a number of interesting trace elements. So there is a lot going on in those little sprouts growing in a tray.

Broccoli plants are a rich source of kaempferol for plant progesterone,[298] and we know they contain lignans, giving you plant estrogen;[299] however, I can't find any studies on the exact amounts of plant hormones in sprouted broccoli, so I can't guarantee numbers on this one. Obviously, broccoli is famous for containing high amounts of glucosinolates, but aside from this, eaten raw, it has lashings of vitamin C, vitamin K, folate, vitamins A and E, a range of B vitamins, and smaller amounts of important minerals such as calcium, magnesium, zinc, phosphorus, and selenium.

Radish sprouts have the highest amount of kaempferol of any of the sprouts that have been tested. They also contain interesting flavonoids, such as morin, myrycetin, and quercetin,[92] which are strong candidates for being progesteronic. Quercetin has been shown to bind to testosterone receptors, so there might be more to radish sprouts than we currently know! I honestly think they are going to be the next big thing in the sprouting world.

Radish also has lashings of cancer-fighting glucosinolates alongside vitamin C, a broad range of B vitamins, vitamin A, and a number of important minerals, such as calcium, magnesium, potassium, iron, and sodium.

Officially, alfalfa has the same hormonal content (isoflavones, coumestrol, and kaempferol) as red clover[92] but in lower amounts. Some people find alfalfa easier to source and grow, so it's a nice backup if you can't get red clover.

Alfalfa contains vitamin K, vitamin C, B complex, vitamin E, calcium, iron, magnesium, potassium, all trace minerals, selenium, and zinc. If you saw all that on a multi-vitamin pill you'd be quite impressed.

Other Reasons to Grow Red Clover, Alfalfa, Broccoli, and Radish Sprouts

There are so many wonderful reasons to grow these sprouted greens that it could be a whole book in itself, so I'll just stick to the highlights!

First off, alfalfa contains saponins, which help push bad fats like LDL cholesterol out of our arteries and increase the HDL good fats! A couple of animal studies [300, 301] and one human study found that you need to take just over a gram of alfalfa sprouts a day. [302] A 6-inch tray of alfalfa will yield around 7 grams, so that's a week's supply.

Other animal studies on alfalfa have shown that it has the potential to treat many autoimmune diseases, including decreasing the severity of lupus.[303] In mice, alfalfa has been shown to have anti-inflammatory activity.[304] It is also great against iron overload [305] but not so good if you are lacking in iron, as it binds to iron and excretes it out of the body.

If I haven't already convinced you to grow red clover for all its plant hormones, then perhaps its effect on diabetes will interest you?[306] Diabetic mice treated with red clover extract for just five weeks showed "significant lowering of blood glucose levels."[307] It is also has proven anti-inflammatory and antioxidant activity.[308] So there are lots of reasons to eat this marvellous sprout, not least because, as mentioned, it has properties that scientists don't understand yet. All they can do is look at the effects and marvel.

There are so many good things about broccoli sprouts that I hardly know where to start. A 2014 study has shown that broccoli sprouts (or the sulforaphane in them) can also help autism. An 18-week double-blind study reported that there was "substantially (and reversibly) improved behaviour compared with 15 placebo recipients." [309] In addition, a 2015 study found that broccoli has the "potential to improve cognitive function in patients with schizophrenia." [310] All of which I find incredible and wonderful. I know this book is about menopause and diseases of aging, but do tell this to anyone you know with an interest in that area.

The wide range of health benefits of broccoli sprouts is probably to do with its power to help the body get rid of toxins. This has now been proven beyond doubt and will affect a whole range of illnesses,[311] including diabetes.[312]

Radish sprouts seem to be the new kid on the block in terms of sprouting, with scientific evidence of their amazing health benefits driving the boom. The truth is that full-grown radishes and their leaves contain excellent nutritional and health-giving qualities, and sprouted radish has 9–59 times the antioxidants of the full-grown plant.[313]

What this means in practice is that radishes have long been known for their cancer-fighting properties.[314] In one study comparing radish and broccoli sprouts, radish sprouts came out better.[315] Tests show radish sprouts can help prevent diabetes[316] and disorders linked to obesity.[317]

Researchers in another study fed radish sprouts to fruit flies for 10 days and found that the sprouts increased their energy and metabolism and lowered their glucose.[318] So if you find yourself troubled by flies getting in your radish sprout trays, you'll know that they have read this study and want to eat them!

Finally, for the aesthetes among you, try growing the sango variety of radish sprouts, as some of the leaves take on a deep red hue. They look absolutely stunning on the plate, and their spicy peppery taste will make your dinner party guests sit up too. Come on, everyone. Let's make radish fashionable again.

CHAPTER 22

How to Grow Fenugreek and Flaxseed (Linseed) Sprouts

Basic Instructions

I have put fenugreek and flax together because they are both sprouts that you can eat at any stage of the sprouting cycle. The only difference in the way you grow them is that you need to soak the flaxseeds overnight before you put them in the tray.

With fenugreek, just sprinkle enough to cover most of the bottom of the sprouting tray, but not so many that they are on top of each other (they are going to double in size so they need room for manoeuvre). Do give them a thorough watering, making sure every seed is wet.

Both flaxseeds and fenugreek get very sticky. Don't worry about it. Let them cling to each other. Flaxseeds grow such wet-looking sprouts, you might not think they need watering, but they do! The good news is that you only need to water flaxseeds and fenugreek twice a day, so you can have a life and your sprouts too! Don't forget: if you are using trays, tip them onto their side to make sure that the water has drained, and don't reuse that water.

Keep trays in indirect sunlight; the warmer it is, the faster they will sprout, but obviously not too hot, as mentioned before. It's a balancing act. Don't put them on a radiator.

Flaxseeds take a few days to start sprouting. Just keep watering, and it will happen. In all, they take 7–9 days to grow to a double leaf. I always have two trays of flaxseeds growing at a time—one to dip into, one still growing; that way I never run out. If the flaxseed tray feels slimy underneath, it means they are going off. Both flaxseeds and fenugreek are happy to grow in stacked trays. Towards the end of the growing cycle, fenugreek sprouts will need to be on top as they become so long they tumble over the side of the tray—looking rather nice, I must say.

ARE FLAXSEEDS DIFFICULT TO SPROUT?

There are a number of sites on the internet that say that flaxseeds are either difficult or impossible to sprout. It is not. It would only be impossible if you use old, dead, hulled, or cooked seed. If you're sure that you are using living flaxseeds, then you can sprout them. They do take a few days longer to get a little white root, so I wonder if people give up and throw them out.

Secondly, make sure you only sprout a thin layer of sprouts, otherwise the ones on top will sprout and the ones underneath will rot.

Thirdly, keep watering and draining them twice a day, even though the stickiness means that they always look wet. Flaxseeds are not your typical sprout, but as you'll see in the next few pages, they are very worth it.

DO I WASH THE HULLS OFF?

Flaxseeds are so healthy, you can eat them without sprouting. The hulls provide lots of fibre, so you don't have to wash them off. In fact, when you grow flaxseeds, by days 4–5 (when they have a long white root) you can eat them directly from the tray; they are very chewy and nice. Eat them before that time, and you'll find they are still too hard.

As I have already mentioned, fenugreek hulls are very pungent, but washing them off does help with this. The best way to get rid of them is to make sure your fenugreek sprouts are grown to double-leaf stage, as many of them will be shed naturally. Then put them in a bowl of water, jiggle them about, and drain. You'll know if you've missed one, though, because of the aroma wafting up from your arm pits. Some people actually like the curry like smell, and if you're one of them, this is a fantastic little sprout.

WHICH VITAMINS, MINERALS, AND PLANT HORMONES DO THEY CONTAIN?

One study found that flaxseeds have roughly 800 times the amount of lignans (plant estrogen) of average plants.[319] That makes them the highest source of plant estrogen anywhere in the known world—more than red clover and more than soya. [320] This was confirmed by another study that found supplementation with flaxseeds produced a greater increase of estrogen in women than soya did.[321]

Flaxseeds also contain a number of flavonols, including our favourite progesteronic, kaempferol. In fact, some flaxseeds are genetically engineered to contain more kaempferol, as a means of enhancing their health benefits.[322] So they are another seed with nicely balanced plant hormones. Flaxseeds are popular subjects for study due to their high lignan, fibre, and oil content.

None of the databases I searched contained data on the nutritional content of flaxseed sprouts. I can tell you that flaxseeds only contain trace amounts of all the main vitamins, but their high mineral content (the most I've seen of any sprout) more than makes up for any shortfall in vitamins. Flaxseeds are high in calcium, iron, magnesium, phosphorus, potassium, manganese, and selenium.

The plant hormones in fenugreek seed sprouts make them potentially the most exciting hormone-balancing food for a menopausal woman to consume. Fenugreek seeds contain isoflavones, lignans, and coumestrol,[323] the three main forms of phytoestrogen, as well as kaempferol and apigenin, and many other flavonols that are possibly progesteronic.[324] More exciting still is that fenugreek seeds also contain diosgenin.[325] You may remember from Part One that diosgenin is the substance in wild yams that scientists convert to progesterone in the laboratory for use in supplements. We now know that our gut bacteria can convert it, too.[96]

I don't know of any other sprouted food that has these three different forms of plant progesterone. In addition, fenugreek seeds contain unique steroidal saponins. First identified in 1952, these steroidal saponins are described as precursors in the synthesis of sex hormones in the body.[326] If scientists eventually discover that there is such a thing as plant testosterone, fenugreek is the top candidate for containing it.

Hearing all this, you start to realize why some people are crazy about fenugreek, especially body builders. There are a number of fenugreek supplements on the market, including Fenusterols® and Testofen (great names, I think!), which both claim to boost testosterone. None of them are cheap, so if you can grow your own, all the better.

If that weren't enough, fenugreek is very high in protein (30 percent) and also contains magnesium, calcium, phosphorus, potassium, sodium, zinc, niacin, iron, arginine, leucine, lysine, aspartic acid, glutamic acid, sulphur, and vitamin E.

OTHER REASONS TO GROW FLAX AND FENUGREEK SEEDS

Herbalists have been using both of these plants for thousands of years. All parts of the flax plant have been used since prehistoric times. The Latin name for flaxseed is *Linum usitatissimum*, the second part of which actually means "very useful." By the way, if you're wondering why I am calling it flaxseed rather than linseed, I have found that, officially, it's flaxseed when used as a food and linseed when used for its fibre and oil. Flax has long been a part of ayurvedic medicine, and is mentioned by Hippocrates in his medical texts.

There are lot of studies on raw flaxseeds, as they are an excellent source of nutrients with anticancer properties, but the seeds alone have limitations on their use because they can cause indigestion and are not readily absorbed during digestion. The problem is that raw flaxseeds contain trace amounts of cyanide, [327] which is why we are encouraged to just have small amounts of them daily or boil them and lose some of the nutritional value.

What is the answer? Well, to sprout them, of course!

I'm not the only one to think this. Even though flaxseed is not known as a typical sprout, bread manufacturers have been commissioning studies to see if adding sprouted flaxseeds would be of more benefit to their consumers, and the results are amazing. One study found that sprouting for just one day led to improvement in nutritional composition—antioxidants doubled, and essential amino acids trebled. It even increased the already abundant lignans! [328]

Fenugreek sprouts are also a powerhouse of nutrients. They are great for blood cleansing, anti-inflammatory, and great for the heart.[329] In addition, numerous studies show that it can be used in the management of diabetes and cancer [330] and can even protect the liver from alcoholic damage. So how about selling fenugreek sprouts in pubs and wine bars? [331] As if that weren't enough, it has been shown to prevent hormonal cancers.[332, 333]

Both fenugreek seeds and leaves have been studied extensively and deemed safe. Folk remedies also have fenugreek as a mouthwash (to cure bad breath), a douche (if you have bacterial problems), and a face cleanser (for acne). So that's all your embarrassing problems solved by one sprout! If you ever have any spare fenugreek sprouts, do run them through your juicer and use the liquid in any way you need to.

CHAPTER 23

How to Grow Cress

Basic Instructions

First, wash your hands (if you are going to handle the food-grade paper). Put a sheet on a flat surface, and wet it. Completely flat plates are best, because the water will graduate towards the centre if there is a rim.

Pour cress seeds directly from the packet onto the paper, or use a spoon. Sprinkle them as evenly as possible, not on top of each other, as they are going to draw water from the paper, so they need to be touching it.

Seeds will stick to the paper within half an hour (you can even hold the plate upside down, and they won't budge). This means that you can pour water directly onto them. Do this gently, though, because if you blast them, they might get dislodged. Some people prefer to spray them. If you do this, always make sure you saturate the paper.

Water whenever the paper dries out, which is more often in the beginning, as the seeds soak it up. Using more than one sheet of food grade paper can cut down on watering, as it holds more. I have used up to three sheets at a time.

Your cress sprouts will be ready when they have a double leaf, usually 5–7 days, depending on the temperature. I keep mine in the dining room in the winter, because they really slow down when it gets cold. When they are ready, put them in a tub in the fridge. They will keep for a week. No need to wash seeds off. Cress seeds have health benefits in their own right.

You can also add other sprouts to your cress mixture. Traditionally, cress seeds were always grown with 25 percent mustard seeds, which I find interesting because they grow at different rates, with cress being the faster seed. I've got around this by soaking the mustard in water overnight beforehand, which gives them a head start.

Some people (including myself) have tried to grow cress in normal sprouting trays, and it just doesn't work. The stickiness clogs the slats, which makes them hard to water, and they come out weedy and sad looking.

WHICH VITAMINS, MINERALS, AND PLANT HORMONES DOES CRESS CONTAIN?

Raw cress is one of the highest sources of kaempferol. It also has other flavonols that are suspected of being progesteronic,[334] so if you're looking for plant progesterone in an easy-to-grow form, this could be the sprout for you. As a bonus it contains plant estrogen in the form of lignans.[42] Garden cress eaten raw contains high amounts of vitamin C, vitamin A, vitamin K, with smaller amounts of a range of B vitamins. In terms of minerals, it is very rich in calcium (which might be why it is so good for bone healing), and contains smaller amounts of magnesium, phosphorus, potassium, and copper.

OTHER REASONS TO GROW CRESS

Put simply, cress is marvellous but deeply out of fashion and overlooked by the sprouting community. [121] We have been eating cress since before written records began, and modern science is proving why. We have already talked about its cancer-fighting, bone-sparing ability, but on top of that it is anti-inflammatory,[335] anti-hypertensive,[336] and has proven useful against both gastrointestinal problems[337] and liver toxicity.[338]

If for any reason you just can't bear the taste of cress, why not put it on your skin? You might be doing this already because a number of cosmetics makers are using cress in their face creams. As one manufacturer stated in its leaflet, "cress sprouts were shown to work as a general anti-aging ingredient by stimulating the cell's own defence system against free radicals."[339] The fact that cress is so easy to grow on food-grade paper means that if you try nothing else in this book, you should at least give cress a go.

GROWING MUSTARD AND OTHER SPROUTS WITH CRESS

As mentioned above, traditionally we used to mix 75 percent cress and 25 percent mustard seed. It works because cress is sticky and keeps the mustard seeds in place; otherwise, they would be washed away when you water them. Reasons to grow cress with mustard seed are that they are another spicy brassica with lots of myrosinase to help our bodies convert health-giving compounds into usable form. Also, uniquely, the cosmetic study mentioned above found that mustard sprouts applied topically to lips boosted their volume.

If your main concern is hormonal health, though, and you don't have time to grow more complicated sprouts such as red clover in trays, adding them to your cress might be a way you can get these sprouts into your life. You could grow your cress with 25 percent red clover, alfalfa, or broccoli; it doesn't have to be mustard. The stickiness of the cress helps the other seeds adhere to paper, too, so this is a wonderful way to combine sprouts for maximum health.

CHAPTER 24

FAQS AND TROUBLESHOOTING

SEEDS THAT WON'T SPROUT

If any of your seeds won't sprout, it could be that they are old. Some seeds spoil easily and won't grow after a couple of years. If I buy seeds in bulk, I store them in the fridge or freezer, and that seems to keep them fresh. I find alfalfa to be a particularly delicate seed.

MOULD

There are three reasons sprouts go mouldy. It might be that you are not draining the trays (just tip them onto their sides) or that you are not watering often enough, or that they are too hot. Again, it's alfalfa that is particularly sensitive to heat. The moment the weather reaches 30 degrees C, they won't grow at all.

Provided you catch mould early enough, you can probably save your sprouts by giving them a long rinse, draining them, and popping them in the fridge for 48 hours. The coolness will kill off the mould, then the sprouts can carry on growing normally. Alternatively, if you are home all day, you can try rinsing the sprouts every 2–3 hours for 24 hours. The constant through-put of water kills mould, too. If your sprouts have turned to slushy mush, there is no saving them I'm afraid!

FLIES

In the height of summer, sprouts do sometimes attract fruit flies. To stop this, tie up sprouting bags, and put lids on your tubs. For green sprouts, I use an empty sprouting tray as my top level, and for cress I put a sieve over them. This is so that the light can still get in, but the flies can't.

WHAT ABOUT HEALTH SCARES?

Every now and then there is a scare about raw sprouts, due to fears about salmonella and E. coli. Salmonella and E. coli are not naturally found in seeds or sprouts and can only get onto them through human contact. If this happens, unfortunately, sprouting trays provide a lovely growing environment, being warm and wet.

I buy most of my seeds (fenugreek, red clover, and broccoli) from specialist sprouting suppliers (see resources) who rigorously test their batches. You don't ever need to touch your sprouts during the growing process. Just pour them into the tray, and water. I do buy mung, lentil, and aduki beans from the health food store, which I sprout and eat raw. I have been eating them raw for 12 years without incident, but we all have to make our own choices. All sprouting seed producers are subject to EU rules and FDA guidance.[340] Seeds have to be both traceable and sampled, so producers have to be extra vigilant these days. You can touch them once they are grown, because you are going to put them in the fridge, where bacteria can't flourish.

Buy all your seeds from specialists, if you want to be sure. The other option is to cook your sprouts. Steaming them is the best option, because it cuts down on the amount of nutrients lost, but does it kill E. coli and Salmonella? In 2010, the American Food and Drug Administration (FDA) looked into this and found that steaming for at least 15 seconds at 72 degrees C (water becomes steam at 100 degrees C) was recommended for killing off potential E. coli bacteria. As for salmonella, I could only find data about steaming chicken skin, but heat does kill salmonella, too.[341] Even cooked, sprouted beans and seeds are healthier than their non-sprouted counterparts, and cooking ensures safety. One company looked specifically at the bacteria on broccoli and radish sprouts and found that they were "below those permitted by legislation (5 mg/100 g of edible food)" and safe to eat.[342]

The other safety issue people ask me about, arose because male sheep in Australia became infertile after grazing on red clover, and everyone was very worried that that might happen to men! Research was rapidly undertaken, and it was found that red clover had absolutely no effect on the males of our species. This is assumed to be because our bodies have evolved eating plant estrogens, whereas the sheep had suddenly had their diet changed from grass to red clover. It was later revealed that it was subterranean clover rather than red clover that had caused the problem.[343]

In fact, the research into the protective effects of plant estrogens on men is very impressive but is outside the scope of this book. So feel free to feed red clover sprouts to everyone you know, regardless of sex.

WHAT'S THE BEST SPROUT FOR ME TO GROW?

If you are struggling time wise, the best sprouts for you to grow are the ones you can fit into your life, the ones your children like watering, and the ones you like the taste of. Personally, I think the perfect trio of sprouts, the loveliest balance of plant estrogens, plant progesterone, and lots of other lovely cancer-preventative plant nutrients is red clover, broccoli, and mung bean sprouts. The three easiest sprouts to grow are mung beans, alfalfa, and cress, and out of those the simplest sprout of all to grow is cress.

WHAT IF YOU REALLY HAVE NO TIME TO GROW THEM?

If you really don't have the time to grow them, then luckily most health food stores sell ready-sprouted alfalfa and mung beans. I have seen other interesting sprout mixes on sale, too, such as radish, broccoli, and red clover. Whether you grow them yourself or get them from the health food store, you are going to get lots of other nutrition from your sprouts. It's not just about phytoestrogens; you are getting a really fresh, fabulous, little, vitamin-packed vegetable, and it might turn you on to the whole idea of sprouting.

HOW MUCH IS SAFE?

Research into safe levels of plant hormones tend to focus on extracts rather than eating the whole plants, but we can still use them as a guide. One study confirmed that "isoflavones consumed orally and in doses below 2 mg/kg body weight per day should be considered safe for most population groups." [344] As I weigh 66kg (146 lb), I can have 132 mg of plant estrogen a day, which seems like a lot.

Another study looking at plant estrogen supplements found no evidence of adverse effects when used for up to two years. [345] This means that if you take supplements, you've got two years to learn how to sprout them instead, because if supplements are safe, the whole plant is going to be even better.

There is also research into how much broccoli sprout extract you can ingest. This is because broccoli has such great cancer-fighting ability that scientists need to know how much they can give people. One study subjected patients to 32 different tests before, during and after giving them high amounts of sprouted broccoli extract and concluded that there were no significant toxic effects. [346] This is marvellous news because the extract is much less natural than eating the whole sprout.

WHAT IF I GET CALLED AWAY OR GO ON HOLIDAY?

If you get called away suddenly and are loath to leave your half-grown trays of sprouts, then just pop them in the fridge. I have left mine for up to five days. They think it's just a cold spell and go into hibernation. Get them out when you get back, water them, and they will burst into to life again. You can, of course, take sprouting bags with you on the road, and hang them up anywhere.

WHAT IF YOU LIVE IN A COUNTRY WHERE YOU CAN'T GET THESE BEANS AND SEEDS?

If you're reading this book in a country where some of the sprouted foods I'm recommending are not easily available, ask yourself what kept your ancestors healthy? What beans are local to your culture? Can you try sprouting them? What vegetables in the brassica family grow where you live?

For example, scientists have tested the roots, seeds, and sprouts of rutabaga (or swede, as we call it here) and found they are fabulous antioxidants with proven anti-cancer effects. [347] However, the sprouting seeds are not available in this country, but they might be where you are.

Similarly, cabbage sprouts have been shown to help prevent Alzheimer's; [348] it's not the kind of cabbage we have in the UK and US, but it might be where you are. A good start is to find out if there is a local sprouting tradition, and also investigate what your great-grandparents ate.

Do all this, and you might even end up writing your own book about it. After all, that's what happened to me!

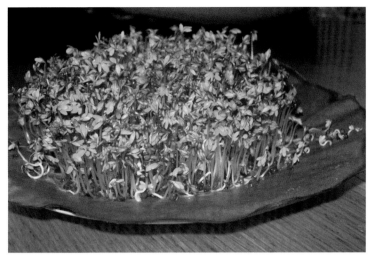

FIG 1: Cress growing on food grade paper, a modern way to bring back an ancient tradition.

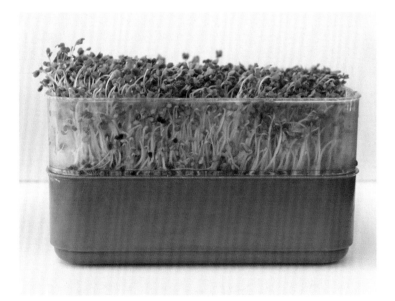

FIG 2: Broccoli sprouts ready to harvest. They don't like to be stacked but you can grow them on the top tray.

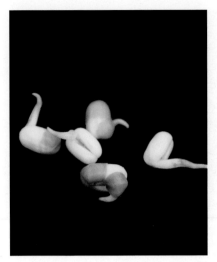

FIG 3: Mung beans – a few days old with a tiny root.

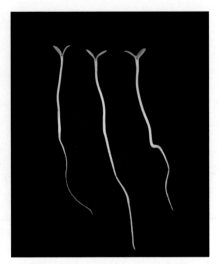

FIG 4: Red clover sprouts, grown to double leaf stage.

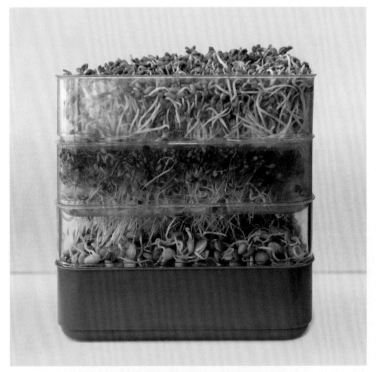

FIG 5: Stack of three trays. Fenugreek growing on top, beans on the bottom, flax in the middle.

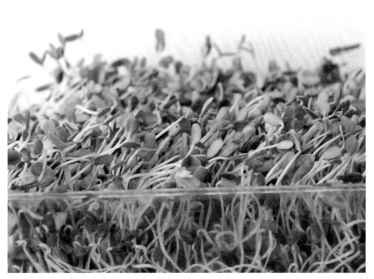

FIG 6: Flax sprouts, absolutely beautiful leaves, full of goodness. They take a bit longer to grow but are worth it.

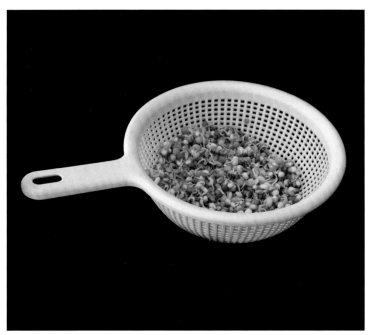

FIG 7: Mung beans and lentil growing in a sieve, a great way to start sprouting.

III

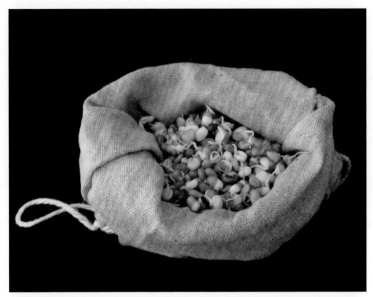

FIG 8: Mung beans in a sprouting bag. You can grow them to a full Chinese style sprout too.

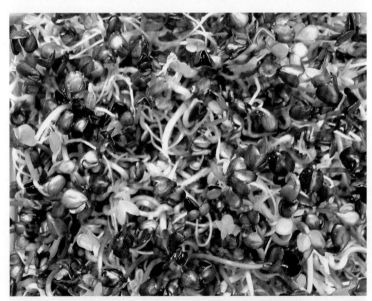

FIG 9: Sango Radish, red and spicy, wonderful for salads.

PART FIVE
– DIGGING DEEPER –

These appendices are for anyone who wants to have a deeper look at some of the things discussed in this book.

The History of Conventional HRT

Many books, scientific studies, research papers, and week-long conferences have taken place on what's right and wrong with traditional HRT, and feelings about it run very high. Basically, if you go on it, you will be given a prescription for hormones extracted from pregnant mares' urine for estrogen, combined with synthetic progesterone.

The history of HRT is very confusing. Some of the earlier studies were so positive about it, doctors called for all menopausal women to be put on HRT immediately. One 1965 scientific study concluded that, "Proof is accumulating that replacement for ovarian failure is beneficial, safe and rewarded by increased health." [349] A 1967 Canadian study, was so sure of how good it was, it included in its title that women "should be treated throughout life by estrogen replacement therapy." [350] Everyone agreed that menopause was caused by ovarian failure and that hormone replacement therapy was the answer.

We know now that those early studies were flawed. They were too small, and in relation to heart disease, they only looked at women who had lower risk factors in the first place. The studies ignored women who couldn't tolerate HRT, which left only the healthier women. One of the main criticisms of the early studies is that they weren't long enough to tease out the real risk factors. [351]

Eventually, some large-scale, long-term studies were started, notably the Wisdom Study, The Million Women Study, [352] and the Women's Health Initiative (WHI).

The Women's Health Initiative Study was dramatically halted after just three years, because the results were so bad it couldn't justify continuing. The WHI study reported that compared to the placebo, estrogen plus synthetic progesterone resulted in increased risk of heart attack, stroke, blood clots, and breast cancer; the only positive was a reduction in the risk of colorectal cancer and fractures. Estrogen taken on its own was slightly better, but previous studies had shown conclusively that this increases the risk of endometrial cancer, so that wasn't a solution, either.

Both the Million Women and Wisdom studies quickly halted, too. The Million Women Study reported that taking HRT increased major cardiovascular disease, osteoporotic fractures, breast cancer, and dementia. It also increased the chances of getting all other cancers, and women on it had a higher death rate generally.[353] None of this looked good, and everyone started speculating about what might be causing the problems.

The late hormone pioneer John Lee, MD, in his book *What Your Doctor May Not Tell You About Menopause*, wrote that the problem might be because the pregnant mares' urine used in the formula has extra molecules that are specific to horses. He pointed out that there has been no research done on what effect they might have on the human body. Moreover, he stated that HRT is given to women in unnaturally high doses that would never occur in nature, and this in itself is a problem.

The tide started to turn against HRT, when it hit the headlines that the studies had been cancelled. Some women literally threw their pills in the bin—only to get them out again a few days later when their symptoms came back with a vengeance. Some women tried to find alternatives to HRT, others tried to "tough it out," or turned to plant hormone supplements, or even menopause cake. Sadly, no one yet knew that you could grow your own hormones. Battles raged in the scientific community about whether HRT was good or bad, and it took 10 years before scientists could properly re-evaluate those studies.

Finally, in 2012, a paper entitled "Have We Come Full Circle—or Moved Forward? "[354] was published on the subject and offered food for thought. It pointed out that the problems with both the WHI and the Million Women study are that they gave HRT to women who didn't have symptoms. Presumably, they did this based on the idea that all menopause is ovarian failure, and that we all need hormone replacement.

As we saw in Part One, we now know that this is not true, so they were basically giving estrogen and progesterone to women who were happily making enough of their own. For these women, extra hormones are obviously a disaster, but, as the re-evaluation points out, for women who do have symptoms it's a completely different matter.

Dr. Alastair H MacLennan,[355] one of the authors of the Wisdom Study, states, "The worse your [menopause] symptoms, the more benefits you get from combined HRT in terms of quality of life, sleep disturbance, physical functioning, and bodily pain."

A second study came to a similar conclusion. It says that a re-analysis of the WHI data "does not justify the continuing negative attitude to HRT in symptomatic women who start HRT near menopause.[356] It turns out that starting and stopping before the age of 60 is crucial in terms of risk factors.

Everyone now agrees that the longer you are on HRT, the higher the risks. The Wisdom Study concluded that it's okay to start taking it in your 50s, but not in your 60s and 70s. Dr. MacLennan further stated that, taken this way, "They have very few risks at all; very few serious morbidities."

Very few, but how many exactly?

Cancer UK has analyzed the statistics based on these results, which makes the costs and benefits clearer. The organization states that "If 1,000 women start taking HRT at the age of 50 for 5 years, two more women get breast cancer and one more gets ovarian cancer." However, it slightly reduces the risk of bowel cancer.

Two in one thousand doesn't sound like very many, as long as it's not YOU! However, because millions of women were taking HRT, even at two cases per thousand, it still added up to a lot of women potentially getting breast cancer from taking traditional HRT.

In 2005, it was announced that as a result of women coming off HRT, "there were 1,400 fewer cases of breast cancer in the UK among women aged 50–59 than would have been." This is correct, but possibly misleading in terms of overall risk. I say "possibly," because a recent study has looked at the figures again and concluded that the breast cancer risk for postmenopausal women on HRT has been underestimated![357]

I'm sure this debate will run and run, but for women over 60, the evidence is more consistent. The BMJ (British Medical Journal) summarized it nicely: breast cancer risk rises to 3–4 cases per 1000, 10 more women will have a stroke, and 5 more will get heart disease.[358]

Even though the message at the moment is to start and stop HRT before the age of 60, Dr. MacLennan believes that older women with continuing symptoms should be assessed on an individual basis, according to risk factors, which are mainly weight, alcohol, family, and personal history. Basically, we all need to make up our own minds. Cancer Research keep a close eye on all research and produce interesting summaries. See more at *www.cancerresearchuk.org*

The good news for HRT is that it does offer some protection from osteoporosis. However, the 2012 Cochrane report stated, "Risk of fracture was the only outcome for which there was strong evidence of clinical benefit from HRT."

But what happens when you come off it? Can you just stop without any symptoms? That will probably depend on the state of your ovaries. If during the time you have been on HRT, the HPA axis (located in the brain and controlling your hormonal needs) has gently settled into retirement and is now asking your ovaries to create fewer hormones, and they are able to respond, then you should have no problem.

One study looked at 1,100 women and found that only 37 percent had their symptoms return after stopping HRT.[359] I couldn't find any data about how long symptoms are likely to last for women for whom they return after stopping HRT. The *Daily Mail's* special "HRT Agony Aunt" (yes, they really do have one)[360] admits that it's hard to say, but symptoms are likely to last about two years. She also says that, in some cases, symptoms are more severe than before the woman started HRT, which is obviously worrying, but it might be about the body rebalancing itself.

So where do you turn when your doctor has no more medicine for you? The HRT agony aunt suggests plant hormones. Some doctors do, too. Given the potential side effects of HRT, having a go at growing your own has got to be worth a try.

Also try looking at other foods you can bring into your diet. Considering the diets that traditional societies eat, we are only being given HRT because we are eating the wrong things anyway. So let's give ourselves a chance to eat the right things. All the evidence is there that it works, and we will get our bodies and hormones back the way mother nature meant them to be.

Supplements: Why the Evidence Is So Contradictory (and What to Do If You Need to Take Them)

In Part One, I talk about how research into supplements is so contradictory. It's almost crazy that whilst some studies find supplements very effective against all menopausal symptoms,[361] others conclude that they don't work at all.[33]

But here's the rub: the Cochrane Collaboration[34] reviewed nearly 50 studies and found that the placebo effect of supplements had up to 59 percent success rate! Good old placebo, eh? The problem is that it means unless the supplements beat that, the study can't claim that they have worked.

I don't think that's the real problem, though. Most of the menopause supplements on the market offer isoflavones that have been extracted from soya beans, red clover, and sometimes alfalfa. In their natural form, these plants all contain three kinds of plant estrogen, not just the isoflavones,[93] whilst red clover and alfalfa have plant progesterone in them, too. [96]

The marketers rarely mention this, though. They like to present facts about the traditional Asian diet and its link to a healthy menopause and old age and imply that if you take an isoflavone supplement you will get the same thing. This overlooks all the other wonderful nutrients and plant hormones that the traditional Eastern diet offers, which won't be appearing in your pill.[362]

Luckily, scientists are starting to separate the effects of foods and pills. A 2003 analysis of 12 studies on soya isoflavones or soya foods found that "Isoflavone preparations seem to be less effective than soya foods."[363] By "soya foods," scientists mean those found in a traditional Japanese diet—the old-fashioned, fermented kind, such as natto, tempeh, and miso, rather than the processed soya we often eat here.

Similarly, the Advertising Standards Authority (ASA) has just upheld a complaint against one supplement maker for advertising the benefits of isoflavone supplement and menopause. One interesting point about the ruling is that they noted that studies on Asian women taking supplements do seem to produce good results, but that might not be relevant to a Western women. Again, this is because the rest of their diet is likely to be more healthy and thus provide other nutrients and plant hormones that help.

Secondly, studies have shown that if you have never eaten soya before, and you suddenly start taking a lot of it, it might actually harm you.[364] This doesn't only apply to menopause symptoms, either; studies into the Japanese low rate of heart disease have concluded that isolated isoflavones alone do not help.[365, 366] However, the traditional Japanese diet does.[367, 368]

The one area where supplements do seem to have a positive effect is if you are at risk of osteoporosis. A Cochrane review looked specifically at isoflavones and bone loss,[369] and concluded that soya isoflavones could help bone formation and prevent osteoporosis.[370] A couple of rat studies have also shown that red clover is also good against bone loss.[371, 372] This is particularly interesting because it mirrors the research into synthetic estrogens (see Appendix 1) in osteoporosis prevention.

So it seems that if you are at risk for this terrible disease and can't get enough plant estrogen in your diet, then you do have options. In fact, many nutritional advisors such as The Women's Nutritional Advisory Service (WNAS) do recommend supplements for Western women who find it hard to adapt their diets sufficiently.

If you are in this situation, look for supplements that contain extracts of whole red clover or alfalfa leaves, so that you will get all the different forms of plant estrogen and other plant nutrients. A review of studies of red clover (rather than soya) found that it may reduce hot flushes, particularly in women with severe symptoms.[373]

The other reason that studies might be inconsistent is that we need gut bacteria to convert plant estrogens into their active form, and none of the earlier research takes this into consideration.[374]

Scientists are now onto this.[375] A 2006 study gave 89 women a mix of soya isoflavones, lactobacilli, magnolia bark extract, vitamin D3, and calcium and got marvellous results, not just for hot flushes but across the whole spectrum of menopausal illnesses, such as insomnia, mood disorders, libido, and dryness problems.[376] It would have been more interesting to see if their vitamin D and magnesium levels were low before they started, because that is a problem in itself. This demonstrates all the other factors at play, and that is why if you can manage to eat healthily you'll have lots less symptoms to start with.

To specifically test the fermenting side of things, a 2016 double-blind study took this on and gave half the women a soymilk drink fermented by lactobacillus (which is how yoghurt is made) and half a placebo. They found that the fermented drink increased the availability of the isoflavones.[377] Supplement makers are realizing this, and some are now adding a probiotic to their mix, which is exciting. They are expensive, though, and you can always take your plant hormones with yoghurt or sauerkraut (and possibly anything else fermented).

It's not just lactobillus, either. A Chinese study of rats also found that bifid bacterium had a similar effect.[378] These bacterial strains can be found in most live natural yoghurts, so don't limit yourself just to lactobillus; we need lots of different strains, so go for variety.

As mentioned earlier, one of the studies found no evidence of adverse effects of supplements when used for up to two years, so that is something.[34] That gives everyone who uses them two years to learn how to grow their own, or find someone else to, or find a way to get them into their life, because if hormones extracted from plants are safe for up to two years, then imagine how wonderful hormones eaten in their natural state will be.

Bioidentical Hormones
(Also Called Bio-Matching or BHRT)

Bioidentical hormones are perceived as more natural than HRT because they have an identical molecular structure as our own hormones. The estrogens are synthesized from the same estrogenic plants and beans I have been talking about: soya, alfalfa, and red clover.

Progesterone is synthesized from wild yam and soya to create what's called "natural" progesterone. Bio-matchers use saliva tests to determine your hormone levels and prescribe an exact dosage, with the aim of getting your hormone levels to that of a younger, menstruating woman. The pharmaceutical industry hates it, of course, and has issued lots of warnings, mainly stating that it lacks evidence. [379]

Industry critics make some interesting points but have put an unnecessarily harsh spin on it. They criticize saliva tests, saying that you should prescribe based upon symptoms alone (which is how HRT is prescribed). I'm sure the bio-matchers aren't ignoring symptoms, and they might be collecting some interesting data that match symptoms with hormone levels, which, personally, I hope one day they will release.

Bio-matchers often use a more gentle form of estrogen called estriol. In Part One, we talked about how estriol is the weakest of all the estrogens and interestingly enough, it is the kind naturally made by postmenopausal women. For that reason, it is seen as more protective. However, at the time of writing, it is banned in America. This was instigated at the request of a pharmaceutical company called Wyeth Pharmaceuticals, which argues that it was "not safe compared to synthetic hormones" (which Wyeth itself markets!) This has provoked a massive backlash. The FDA has received a record number of complaints and there is a big campaign called "Save our Hormones."

In the meantime, estriol is still available in Europe and Asia, while studies on bio-matching are slowly coming through. A 2013 study of 75 women on estriol has produced favourable results.[380] It reported that menopausal symptoms were "significantly relieved" by estriol, and that "cardiovascular biomarkers, inflammatory factors, immune signalling factors, and health outcomes were favourably impacted." However, despite calling itself a long-term study, it only lasted 36 months, and as we have seen from the history of hormone replacement, that isn't nearly long enough.

Another study undertaken by a community pharmacy lasted seven years, but sadly, it only looked at 200 women, and followed each patient for just three months, with a six-month follow up.[381]

I hope new research will be available soon. The International Menopause Societies guidelines do not recommend bio-matching, although they do endorse natural progesterone, which is available over the counter in the USA but only on prescription in the UK. As we have seen in Chapter 7, there is lots of evidence that it is safer than the synthetic version. It is estimated that up to 2.5 million American women aged 40 years or older use bioidentical hormone therapy.[382]

The main problem I can see with bio-matching is that compounding pharmacies and companies selling the product over the counter are still extracting, isolating, and synthesizing natural hormones, so what they offer is still fundamentally drug based. They are working with their current understanding of hormones, which is not yet comprehensive and might never be. We haven't identified all of the plant chemicals that exist and how they interact with our hormonal systems, and we certainly don't know how they all work together.

Of course, I don't want you to do bio-matching; I want you to grow your own hormones. But if I had to choose between bio-matching and HRT, I would go for bio-matching, not least because they use natural progesterone.

The other downside of bio-matching is that it is very expensive. Radio 4 reported that a listener paid one company £250 for a first consultation, plus £700 for tests. That's without prescribing any medicine.[383]

However, its advocates have been wowed by it. If you have serious menopause problems, are not worried about the cost, and need a quick solution their approach might be right for you.

The Hard Evidence About Endocrine-Disrupting Chemicals in the Environment

There are so many studies about the harmful effects of xenestrogens or endocrine-disrupting chemicals (EDCs) it is impossible to overestimate the problem.

To give you an idea of the scale, what follows is a selection of scientists' conclusions—in their own words.

To understand what these studies are saying you need to understand a few terms.

- Anovulation – not ovulating
- Ocylite – an egg.
- Steroidogenesis – the creation of hormones
- Epigenetics – the study of changes in organisms caused by modification of gene expression rather than alteration of the genetic code itself

A 2011 report from the University of Illinois discussed the widespread impact of EDCs on our ovaries and hormonal signalling:

Disruptions in ovarian processes by EDCs can lead to adverse outcomes such as anovulation, infertility, estrogen deficiency, and premature ovarian failure among others ... They interfere with hormone signalling via two mechanisms: altering the availability of ovarian hormones, and altering binding and activity of the hormone at the receptor level. Among the chemicals covered are pesticides (e.g. dichlorodiphenyltrichloroethane and methoxychlor), plasticizers (e.g. bisphenol A and phthalates), dioxins, polychlori-

*natedbiphenyls, and polycyclic aromatic hydrocarbons (e.g. ben-
zo[a]pyrene).[384]*

A 2014 report published in the Journal of the Institute of Experimental
Endocrinology shows that ovarian hormones are being targeted by EDCs,
and industrial chemicals are being found in ovaries of women.

> *(We) report that ovarian steroid hormone production is being recog-
> nized as an important target for the action of endocrine disrupting
> chemicals (EDCs). The fact that these chemicals have been detected
> in the biological samples of general population, and even directly in
> the follicular fluid of women, emphasizes the demands for testing
> the influence of EDCs on ovarian steroidogenesis.[385]*

A 2008 report by Maryland college in Tennessee offers an overview of how
EDCs cause reproductive disorders and how this can be passed on to the
next generation.

> *This study provides an overview of the human epidemiological
> evidence documenting the detrimental effects of several common
> environmental EDCs on female reproduction. We then focus on
> experimental evidence demonstrating the epigenetic effects of these
> EDCs in the ovary and female reproductive system, with an empha-
> sis on methoxychlor, an organochlorine pesticide.[386]*

A 2012 report by the State University of New Jersey argues that our reproductive systems are at particular risk if exposed to EDCs in early life.

> *The data reviewed illustrates that EDCs contribute to numerous
> human female reproductive disorders and emphasize the sensitivity
> of early life-stage exposures…*
> *Epidemiological studies strongly suggest that EDCs affect both male
> and female reproduction.[387]*

This is from the same university, warning that disruptive effects can pass
from one generation to the next.

Importantly, EDCs that can directly target the ovary can alter epigenetic mechanisms in the oocyte, leading to transgenerational epigenetic effects. [388]

Just to give you a flavour of some of the scary stuff around plastic, a study by Yale University states that EDCs:

Have effects on male and female reproduction, breast development and cancer, prostate cancer, neuro-endocrinology, thyroid, metabolism and obesity, and cardiovascular endocrinology. [389]

And if you don't believe me, try this quote from Tulane University's Department of Endocrinology teaching material.

Chemicals used in household and industrial detergents ... can cause an estrogen-like response at the wrong time or in the wrong amounts in both sexes. These kinds of estrogen mishaps can enhance female traits in males (feminize) or cause permanent birth defects that jeopardize survival and reproduction. In addition, kepone and o,p'-DDD can block progesterone receptors on the outside membrane layer of sperm cells, preventing them from becoming competent to fertilize eggs. [390]

And if you're wondering why they're referring to EDCs (Endocrine Disrupting Compounds) rather than a specific hormone, it's because studies find that it's not just estrogen receptors that these chemicals were disrupting; it was our progesterone and thyroid hormones, too.

Why Haven't Chemical and Industrial Hormone Mimics Been Banned?

In the face of overwhelming evidence about the effects of hormone-disrupting chemicals in the environment, you might wonder how the chemical industry still manages to argue against them being banned.

The answer is by getting very creative indeed. Firstly, the chemical industry has produced its own formula by which it measures whether a certain chemical can cause harm, then it pronounces that by that definition, its chemicals are safe.[391] This formula argues that for a chemical to be harmful, it has to have a bad effect on *every* person it comes in contact with.

World Health Organization (WHO) scientists responded by pointing out that by that definition, you could conclude that smoking doesn't cause lung cancer, because not everyone who smokes dies of it.

Secondly, scientists working for the chemical industry try to present industrial hormones pesticides and fungicides as natural. They do this by putting them in the same category as plant hormones—yes, those lovely plant hormones that I have spent this book trying to get you to grow!

They argue that because plant estrogens have an effect on our hormone receptors, they are also "hormone disruptors"; it doesn't matter that they affect them in a positive way. It's a brilliant strategy. Once they have got plant hormones and industrially produced hormones in the same bracket, they can say that our bodies know how to excrete plant hormones, so they must know how to excrete chemical and industrial hormones

They say we evolved on plant hormones, so we must be able to cope with chemical and industrial hormones.

They point to studies showing that gorillas and monkeys eat lots of plant hormones in the jungle so therefore it is fine for humans to be exposed to industrial and chemical hormones.

Reporting on an ape/plant hormone study,[129] *New Scientist* magazine said: "Interest in how primates respond to estrogen disruptors has been sparked by the rising levels of synthetic estrogenic chemicals in our environment, such as bisphenol A, although Wasserman [the study author] cautions that these synthetic forms might act differently from the natural versions."[392]

I nearly shouted at the page when I read that! Of course, synthetic hormones are different from plant hormones. We have already seen both the damage that chemical hormones do and how populations who consume high amounts of plant hormones have lower rates of cancer, osteoporosis, heart problem, strokes, and dementia.

Other scientists argue that because we evolved on plant hormones, we share "an intimate and ancient co-evolutionary history" and that our bodies actually rely on them.[128] We have special receptors on our cells designed to fit specific hormones, just as a key fits a lock, which is the ultimate proof that our bodies need them.[80] Furthermore, the body knows how to excrete plant hormones through urine, whereas industrially produced hormones get stored in our body tissues.

As a result, some eminent scientists are now calling for natural plant and industrially produced hormones to be renamed.[393] My favourite suggestion for what we should call plant estrogens is archiestrogens.[394] It means "ancient estrogens," (in other words, naturally occurring), and that separates them beautifully from the modern synthetic stuff. It's so obvious that we need to differentiate between plant hormones, which are good for us, and industrial hormones, which can be so bad.

If I am sounding very biased, I'm in good company. Over and over, WHO scientists point to evidence that "clearly [shows] that industrial chemicals interfere with hormone action in ways that cannot be considered similar to natural environmental stressors and are often irreversible."[395,396]

I'm going to say it again: chemical and industrial hormones are upsetting our ovaries, giving us early menopause with lots of horrible symptoms, and contributing to the diseases of aging. Whereas, as we have seen, plant hormones are very much part of the solution.

No matter how much evidence WHO scientists provide, though, the chemical industry keeps arguing. WHO scientists are now getting exasperated and have publicly stated that they don't think the chemical industry is even interested in having a scientific debate; what they want is to influence politicians and policy makers.[397]

And that's probably as near the truth as we can get.

As consumers, we can join this argument and vote with our choices and our wallets. We can choose to avoid these chemicals as much as possible, especially those in cosmetics and toiletries. Chapter 17 will show you how.

LIST OF ESTROGENIC FOODS

There are a number of databases I could choose from to compile a list of estrogenic foods. Such is the marvelousness of science, there is even a database of databases! [398]

Here's the rub though. Because different foods are grown from different seeds in different environments, they all give slightly different figures. So take my chart as a rough guide.

I have primarily used a 2009 British study [399] as the basis for this list, not just because I'm patriotic but because it includes all three main types of phytestrogens (isoflavones, lignans, and coumestrol) and is fairly recent. I also used a 2006 Canadian study [93] for any foods I thought should have been included but weren't there, such as squash nuts and seeds.

Most of the data found in the British and Canadian databases were similar. The exception was garlic, which differed from 99ug/100g in British garlic compared with a massive 603ug/100g in Canadian garlic. A third source—Anderson and Sarwar, see below—put garlic at 379ug, so I have averaged garlic in this table to 360ug.

Sadly, lots of the sprouted foods we are interested in did not appear in the standard databases because they are not considered common enough. So I have gone directly to individual studies for these figures and have put my sources below. All foods are in ugs per 100g. Ugs are micrograms; 1,000 ug makes a milligram (mg).

None of the databases included red clover as it is considered to be a herb rather than a food. So I took the red clover stats from other sources. [400] The statistics for avocados also vary drastically. The SWAN phytoestrogen database says they have a massive 400ug of lignans, [401] while the Canadian database puts them at zero! Chung-ja et al come in the middle with 92ugs. [402] So I have gone with that one.

Food per 100g	Total Plant Estrogen Content	Isoflavones Ug per 100g	Lignan Ug per 100g	Coumestrol Ug per 100g
Flaxseeds (linseeds)	379012	321	375321.9	46.8
Tofu (soya bean curd)	27150	27118.5	30.9	0.7
Soya beans (cooked)	17556	175441	11	2
Soya yoghurt	10275	10228	47	
Sesame	8008.1	10.5	7997	
Flaxseed bread	7540.6	300.8	7239	0.6
Red clover	7328.8	7000	44.8	280
Alfalfa sprouts	3100	1,500		46.8
Chickpea sprouts	1600	1600		
Chickpea paté	1493	1444	49	
Dates (dried)	589	14	584	1
Mung bean sprouts	495.1	229.8.	128.7	136.6
Apricots (dried)	443	12	431	1
Broccoli (raw)	437		437	
Chickpeas (cooked)	421	416	4	1
Figs	389	12	376	1
Pistachios	376	177	199	7
Prunes (dried)	363	6	357	1
Garlic	360	2	358	-
Pomegranate	304	304	-	-
Prune (semi-dried)	284	3	281	
Chestnuts (cooked)	283	2	280	1
Sweet potato	259	1	258	
Blackberries (stewed)	221	1	220	1
Chestnuts	217	2	214	1
Brown sauce	215	46	168	1
Parsley	197	59	137	1
Dates (Medjool)	193	35	157	1
Olive oil	180.7	38	142.6	0.1
Chickpea hummus	170	135	34	1
Dates (Deglet - boxed)	168	4	163	1

Food per 100g	Total Plant Estrogen Content	Isoflavones Ug per 100g	Lignan Ug per 100g	Coumestrol Ug per 100g
French beans	159	48	109	2
Runner beans	156	132	18	7
Asparagus (cooked)	154	2	152	
Plum (yellow-cooked)	152	2	150	
French beans (raw)	147	50	94	3
Haricot Beans	132	21	106	5
Almonds	130.5	18	112	1.5
Figs (dried)	129	14	114	1
Carrots (raw)	125	4	121	1
Gooseberries (stewed)	123	1	121	1
Cashews	122	22	99	1
Carrots (cooked)	114	3	111	
Winter squash	113		113	
Kiwi (peeled)	111		111	
Blackcurrants (fresh)	110	2	107	1
Prunes (cooked)	108	2	106	
Hazelnuts	107	30	77	
Green beans	106	39	67	
Peaches (medium)	106	4	102	
Greengages	105	2	103	
Cauliflower	97		97	
Broccoli (cooked)	96	3	90	3
Red wine (6oz glass)	94	29	65	
Cabbage	93		93	
Avocado	92		92	-
Cranberries	92	3	88	1
Raisins	87	17	70	
Peanut butter	79	42	37	
White beans	73	39	34	
Gooseberries (raw)	72	1	71	
Passion fruit	70	43	26	2

Food per 100g	Total Plant Estrogen Content	Isoflavones Ug per 100g	Lignan Ug per 100g	Coumestrol Ug per 100g
Spring onions	62	9	53	
Apricots (stoned)	52	1	52	
Marrowfat peas (tinned)	51	50	1	
Watercress	46	1	45	
Lentils (dried)	36.5	9.5	26.6	0.3
Plums (yellow – raw)	26	2	24	

The broccoli, cabbage, and cauliflower stats are also from Chung-Ja et al. The chickpea stats come from a study that sprouted then dried them, which reduced 50g of sprouts to 25g of extract, thus concentrating the amount twofold. For this reason, I have halved their results. Sadly, they didn't count all eight of the different forms of phytestrogen that chickpeas contain, but the results are still impressive. [281]

LIST OF PROGESTERONIC FOODS

Even though the research into plant progesterone is new, research into kaempferol and apigenin is not, so I do have a list of plants for you.

This database is in mg per 100g, so the figures you see are 100 times stronger than the plant estrogen database, which makes it easier to get plant progesterone if you eat the right foods.

Food	Kaempferol Content Mg per 100g	Apigenin Content Mg per 100g
Capers	135.56	
Parsley	1.49	302
Cumin	38.6	
Mustard greens	38.3	Exact amount unknown [404]
Celery		33.8
Kale (raw)	26.74	
Cloves	23.8	
Radish sprouts (raw)	21.85	
Bell pepper		27.2
Kumquats raw		21.87
Garlic		21
French peas (petits pois)		17.6
New Zealand spinach (this variety only)		15
Garden cress (raw)	13	
Chia seeds (raw)	12.3	
Watercress (raw)	10	

Food	Kaempferol Content Mg per 100g	Apigenin Content Mg per 100g
Chives (raw)	10	
Juniper Berries		5.57
Cherry tomatoes	6.67	
Broccoli (raw)	6.16	
Cress (raw)	4.1	
Sage/Oregano/Marjoram		2.4 – 4.4
Raisins, golden seedless	2.71	
Horseradish	2.57	
Cherries, sour dry unsweetened	3.60	
Broccoli (cooked)	1.38	
Kiwi Fruit	1.03	
Brussels sprouts, raw	0.95	
Gooseberries (raw)	.88	
Radishes (raw)	0.86	
Alfalfa sprouts (raw)	0.86	
Mustard greens (cooked)	0.84	
Red clover (raw)	0.80	
Strawberries (raw)	0.79	
Currents european (raw)	0.71	
Apricots (raw)	0.63	
Rutabagas/swedes (raw)	0.57	
Strawberries (frozen, unsweetened)	0.53	
Beans (snap, yellow - raw)	0.42	
Beans (snap, green – raw)	0.41	
Chinese cabbage (bok choi - raw)	0.37	18.7
Broad beans/fava beans (tinned)	0.35	
Onions (cooked, boiled, drained, without salt)	0.35	
Tea (instant, unsweetened, powder - prepared)	0.32	
Watercress (steamed)	0.27	
Beans (snap, green, frozen, cooked)	0.26	

Food	Kaempferol Content Mg per 100g	Apigenin Content Mg per 100g
Cauliflower (raw)	0.25	
Beans (snap, green, frozen, all styles, unprepared)	0.24	
Cherries, sweet, raw	0.24	
Peaches	0.22	
Radish sprouts	0.22	
Onions (raw)	0.18	
Cabbage (raw)	0.12	
Apricot jams and preserves	0.11	
Cranberries (raw)	0.09	
Tomato products (tinned puree)	0.08	
Blackberries (raw)	0.08	
Iceberg lettuce (raw)	0.07	.38
Tomatoes (red, ripe, raw, year-round average)	0.07	
Spinach (raw)	0.01	
White table wine, beer, alcoholic beverage (average)	0.01	4.17 (beer only)

Like my estrogen list, I cannot find figures for some of the sprouted foods that we know are rich in progesterone. This is because databases often look at common foods, and sprouted foods sadly are not (yet!) common. Fenugreek is missing. Germinated fenugreek contains high amounts of apigenin and smaller amounts kaempferol,[94] as well as unknown amounts of diosgenin,[403] which possibly makes it the most progesteronic of all!

Neither can I find the stats for sprouted broccoli or mustard; only for the full-grown plant or the seed. All of the evidence indicates that sprouting increases phytochemicals, which should mean that sprouted broccoli and mustard have more kaempferol (as their cousin, the sprouted radish, does), but until a study specifically looks at that, I can't add it officially to my database. Also, as with the phytoestrogens, statistics vary wildy from database to database, so take this as a rough guide. I think the one thing all the databases agree on is that a wide variety of fruits and vegetables contain lots of different wonderful compounds. Unless otherwise stated statistics are from *www.nutrition.merschat.com*. I love this online database because it is easily searchable and it references where it gets its stats from.

Raw garden cress, raw chives, steamed watercress, parsley, mustard greens, apricots, and radish sprouts statistics came from USDA database, *Flavonoid Content of Selected Foods, Release 3.1* (2014)

Cress sprouts are not in the standard databases, but luckily a 2013 study looked at all the flavonoids in sprouted cress. To do this they freeze-dried it, which takes roughly 90 percent of the water out of it. So I have taken just 10 percent of the figure they estimated, which was 41mg/g (410mg/100g).[405]

Red clover was not included in either database. The figure I have quoted is for red clover blossom, specifically *Trifolium pratense* (used for sprouting and menopausal symptoms).[406]

Alfalfa statistics are from Janicki et al.[92]

Apigenin stats are from Koo et al.[407] apart from the herbs, which come from Zheng et al.[408]

Cloves and cumin were from Shan et al.[409]

Cherry tomatoes were from Stewart et al.[410]

Resources and Interesting Sites

My Website

Growyourownhrt.com
I will be posting more of my menopause diary and maybe some recipes and articles updating any new science that comes in on this topic. I do sell a few things, where there are gaps in the market. At present, you can buy some sprouting seeds, food-grade paper, and a cress-growing kit.

Specialist Seeds and Beans - UK

Sky Sprouts
Totnes,
Devon,
TQ9 7LP
www.skysprouts.co.uk

Aconbury Sprouts
Courtlands, Allensmore
Hereford, HR2 9AB
Tel: (01432) 360 935
www.wheatgrass-uk.com

Specialist Seeds and Beans - USA

Sprout People
170 Mendell St.
San Francisco, CA 94124
www.sproutpeople.org/seeds

Sproutman
PO Box 1100,
Great Barrington, MA 01230
www.sproutman.com

The Sprout House
874 Neighborhood Road
Lake Katrine, NY 12449
www.sprouthouse.com

BIBLIOGRAPHY

There aren't many books in my bibliography, as I went directly to the scientific papers for my research.

If I had to pick one book for the serious menopause reader it would be the late Dr. John Lee's book (co-written with Virginia Hopkins, who continues Dr. Lee's work today). Although the book was written way back in 1995, Dr. Lee's knowledge of women's bodies, menopause problems, and their causes is impressive. He was way ahead of his time. I learnt so much from him. His book is a classic.

Bown, Stephen R. *The Age of Scurvy*. Chichester, West Sussex, UK: Summersdale. 2003.

Bryson, Bill. *At Home: A Short History of Private Life*. London: Black Swan/Penguin Random House UK. 2011.

Carson, Rachel. *Silent Spring*. London: Hamish Hamilton/Penguin Random House UK. 1963.

Fallon, Sally with Mary Enig, PhD. *Nourishing Traditions*. White Plains, MD: New Trends Publishing Inc. 2009.

Greer, Germain. *The Change: Women, Ageing, and the Menopause*. London: Penguin Books. 1992.

Glenville, Marilyn. *Natural Solutions to Menopause*. Emmaus, PA: Rodale. 2013.

Korach, Kenneth S. ed. *Reproductive and Developmental Toxicology*. Boca Raton, FL: CRC Press. 1998.

Lee, John and Hopkins, Virgina. *What Your Doctor May Not Tell You About Menopause*. New York: Grand Central Publishing. 2005.

Murray, Jenni. *Is It Me, Or Is It Hot In Here?* London: Vermilion/Penguin Random House UK. 2003.

Wilson, Robert. *Feminine Forever.* London: W. H. Allen/Penguin Random House UK. 1966.

List of Photos
(Colour Insert, Pages I to IV)

FIG 1: Cress on food grade paper
FIG 2: Broccoli sprouts in tray
FIG 3: Young mung beans
FIG 4: Red clover
FIG 5: Fenugreek, flax and beans in stack of trays
FIG 6: Flax sprouts
FIG 7: Mung beans and lentil in sieve
FIG 8: Mung beans in sprouting bag
FIG 9: Sango Radish

Acknowledgements

If you are going to lock yourself away for a few years to research a science book, then you need the following:

A really good neighbour, who pops in to see you, walks around the park with you, gives you a break from the science with top chat about boyfriends, beauty, food, and local gossip. I am honoured to have met Angie Cornelius. We've laughed, we've cried, we've lunched! Thank you, darling.

You also need a number of other really close friends who phone up, meet up, or visit regularly and will even read your manuscript, despite being really busy themselves. My little gang consists of the following brilliant women: Jenny Allen, Sue Middleton, and Tessa Levy. Thank you, girls.

Next you need lovely friends who can also chat though all the nutritional and other hormonal aspects with you. Thanks to Jacqui Campbell, who also fed me some of the most superb food I've ever tasted. Plus Paris Nolan and Gary Rolf, who shared their unique take on hormones over delightful cups of tea and walks around the park.

Of course you need to test your menopause theory on real women. Luckily for me, a few brave souls stepped forward, took away sprouting trays and seeds, and shared every detail of their reproductive cycles with me. I am immensely grateful to Kate Tym, Joanne Edwards, Viryapuspa Nolan, and Lisa Harman Pope for growing and eating sprouted foods and writing the diaries published in this book.

It is all very well looking at science papers and researching theories, but it gets to the point where you need a real scientist to talk to. Luckily for me I am friends with the brilliant Dr. Richard Marton, who took up the challenge. Not only did he read my manuscript and offer insightful comments, he did a nice line in general chat, too. I can't thank you enough.

Once the book is well underway, you need lots of general readers to give you feedback and comments, or simply to let you know that what you are doing might be of interest to someone. So big thanks, friends and family—Sue Grella, Angie McAvoy, Simon Dowd, Jean Kelley, Suz Evasdaughter, Trevor Goodwin (who also came up with the sub-title), Lynsey Duffell, and Jeanette Tuck.

Just when you are wondering who is going to help you do the final proofread, you need a couple of old friends to casually comment on how great they are at spotting typos and then agreeing to read a menopause book, despite being in the comedy business. I am hugely grateful to Andrew Jobbins and Maureen Younger for taking up the task—Thank you both so much.

You also need not one but two writers groups to absorb your output (or I did). Firstly, Performers Who Write, whose members at various times consisted of Sheila Hyde, Lisa Harman Pope, Kate Tym, John Knowles, Jonathon Broughton, Mike Hatchard, Rob Hill, and Carol Prior. Secondly, my women's writers group, consisting of Suz Evasdaughter, Viryapuspa Nolan, Angie Cornelius, and Fiona Smith.

Special mention to Sheila Hyde and Suz Evasdaughter, for always telling me when something wasn't working, which meant when they said they liked something, I was thrilled. Particular thanks, Suz, for stepping in at the last minute, reading large chunks of the book, and giving me both speedy turnaround and spot-on comments—this is a better book for you having read it.

Then you need a great photographer to take beautiful stills of the individual sprouts (not as easy as it sounds), get the trays of greens in the right light, and find a setting that makes you look both your real age, yet interesting and lovely. So a huge thank you to Bea Lacey.

None of this book would have been possible without the internet. I am grateful to the scientists who publish their work freely, especially those who allow full access to laypeople like myself. The scientific evidence behind this book is all down to them. I feel profound gratitude. I did have qualms about quoting so many studies done on rats. So thank you, rats, and I'm sorry that things are this way.

This book would also not have happened without all the years I spent growing, experimenting, and talking about sprouted foods with Mr. Steve Savage. This book is for you, too.

Thanks also to Stephen R. Bown, who has given me permission to quote copiously from his book *The Age of Scurvy*. His research helped me expound on how similar the scurvy and menopause stories are.

I am grateful to my editor, Nicky Leach at Findhorn Press, for insightful comments and fine attention to detail. This has made my book both deeper and more readable than I could have managed on my own. Thank you.

I am lucky to have a fantastic dog to walk around the park, allowing time for all the ideas to ruminate in my head. So thank you, Muffin, my little companion. May you long be by my side.

And finally, we all need a guardian angel, someone who looks out for you, sometimes near, sometimes far. I would like to thank mine from the bottom of my heart.

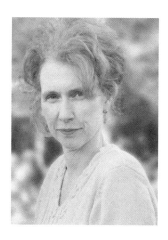

About the Author

Sally J. Duffell is a unique combination of scientific investigator, ex-stand-up comic and bean sprouting expert.

She has been growing, teaching and writing about bean sprouting for many years, and has now extensively researched the scientific proof behind their rich bounty of plant hormones and their effects on menopause symptoms and the diseases of aging. Challenging the traditional view of menopause, Sally revives an ancient, natural way of preventing hot flushes, and other signs of aging, that is simple and easy to do.

For more information see her website: *www.growyourownhrt.com*

END NOTES

1   Michael Gurven and Hillard Kaplan. Longevity Among Hunter- Gatherers: A Cross-Cultural Examination. Population and Development Review. 2007

2   Spitzer, D. Centre for the Cross-Cultural Study of Health and Healing, Department of Anthropology, University of Alberta 1994

3   Caspari, R and Lee, SH. Older age becomes common late in human evolution. Proc Natl Acad Sci U S A. 2004

4   Margaret Walker and James Herndon. Menopause in Nonhuman Primates? Biology of Reproduction. 2008

5   Dr Ronald Lee of the University of California at Berkeley, writing in the journal, Proceedings of the National Academy of Sciences. 2003

6   Cooper RL, Conn PM and Walker RF. Characterization of the LH surge in middle aged female rats. Biol Repred. 1980

7   Jenni Murray, *Is it me, or is it hot in here.* 2001 Vermillion (imprint of Ebury Publishing) – Page 27

8   John Lee, (with Victoria Hopkins). *What your doctor might not tell you about the menopause.* 1996 Little Brown and Company. Page 154

9   Currier, Andrew. F. A consideration of the Phenomena Which Occur to Women, at the Close of the Child-Bearing Period, with Incidental Allusions to Their Relationship to … (Especially the Artificial) Menopause 1897

10   Cook, Frederick . A study of the sexual peculiarities of the American Indian women." I could not find the original book but he is quoted in Andrew Curriers book (referenced above) that was written in 1897, so this study must predate that.

11   Martin MC, Block JD, Sanchez SD, et al. Menopause without symptoms: the endocrinology of menopause among rural Mayan Indians. Maturitas. Am J Obstet Gynecol. 1983

12   Mcewen D C. Ovarian failure and the menopause. Can Med Assoc J. 1965

13   Keettel WC and Bradbury JT. Premature ovarian failure, permanent and temporary. Am J Obstet Gynecol. 1964

14   Hall JE, Lavoie HB, Marsh EE and Martin KA. Decrease in gonadotropin-releasing hormone (GnRH) pulse frequency with aging in postmenopausal women. J Clin Endocrinol Metab. 2000

15   Jodi L. Downs and Phyllis M. Wise. The role of the brain in female reproductive aging. Mol Cell Endocrinol. 2008

16 Janet E. Hall. Neuroendocrine Changes with Reproductive Aging in Women. Semin Reprod Med. 2007

17 Yin W and Gore AC. Neuroendocrine control of reproductive aging: roles of GnRH neurons. Reproduction. 2006

18 Neal-Perry G, Nejat E and Dicken C. The neuroendocrine physiology of female reproductive aging: An update. Maturitas. 2010

19 Aschheim P. Results Provided by Heterochronic Grafts of the Ovaries in the Study of the Hypothalamo-Hypophyso-Ovarian Regulation of Senile Rats. Gerontologia.1964

20 Peng MT, Huang HH. Aging of hypothalamic-pituitary-ovarian function in the rat. Fertil Steril. 1972

21 Wise PM, Smith MJ, Dubal DB, et al. Neuroendocrine modulation and repercussions of female reproductive aging. Recent Prog Horm Res. 2002

22 Greenblatt RB, Natrajan PK and Tzingounis V. Role of the hypothalamus in the aging woman. J Am Geriatr Soc. 1979

23 Parker WH, Broder MS, Chang E, et al. Ovarian conservation at the time of hysterectomy and long-term health outcomes in the nurses' health study. Obstet Gynecol. 2009

24 Parker WH, Broder MS, Liu Z, et al. Ovarian conservation at the time of hysterectomy for benign disease. Clin Obstet Gynecol. 2007

25 Parker WH. Ovarian conservation versus bilateral oophorectomy at the time of hysterectomy for benign disease. Menopause.2014

26 Greer, G, *The Change: Women, Aging and the Menopause*, (1991). Hamish Hamilton Ltd. Page 5

27 Lock, M. *Encounters with Aging: Mythologies of Menopause in Japan and North America*, Berkeley: University of California Press, 1993

28 Lock M, Kaufert P. Menopause, local biologies, and cultures of aging. Am J Hum Biol. 2001

29 Adlercreutz, H. Western diet and Western diseases: Some hormonal and biochemical mechanisms and associations. Scand J Clin Lab Invest Suppl. 1990

30 Wu AH, Ziegler RG, Horn-Ross PL, et al. Tofu and risk of breast cancer in Asian-Americans. Cancer Epidemiol Biomarkers Prev. 1996

31 Dean Houghton, writing for The Furrow Magazine, published by John Deere

32 Kronenberg F, Fugh-Berman A. Complementary and alternative Medicine for menopausal symptoms: review of randomized, controlled trials. Ann Intern Med. 2002

33 Vesco KK, Haney E, Fu R, Nedrow A, et al. Nonhormonal therapies for menopausal hot flashes: systematic review and meta-analysis. JAMA. 2005

34 Lethaby A, Marjoribanks J, Kronenberg F, et al. Phytestrogens for menopausal vasomotor symptoms. Cochrane Database Systematic Review. 2013

35   Ward WE and Thompson LU. Dietary Estrogens of plant and fungal origin occurrence and exposure. p 104. *Handbook of Environmental Chemistry*. Edited by Metzler. 2001

36   Fox, Barthold, Davisson, Newcomer, Quimby and Smith (editors) The Mouse in Biomedical Research: Normative Biology, Husbandry, and Models 2007 p 349

37   Bishnoi S, Khetarpaul N andYadav RK. Effect of domestic processing and cooking methods on phytic acid and polyphenol contents of pea cultivars (Pisum sativum). Plant Foods Hum Nutr. 1994

38   Horn-Ross PL, Hoggatt KJ and Lee MM. Phytestrogens and thyroid cancer risk: the San Francisco Bay Area thyroid cancer study. Cancer Epidemiol Biomarkers Prev. 2002

39   Mira Soni, Tri Budi W. Rahardjo, et al. Phytestrogens and cognitive function: A review. Maturitas. 2014

40   D'Adamo CR and Sahin A. Soy foods and supplementation: a review of commonly perceived health benefits and risks. AlternTher Health Med. 2014

41   Calderón-Montaño JM, Burgos-Morón E, Pérez-Guerrero C, et al. A Review on the Dietary Flavonoid Kaempferol. Mini Rev Med Chem. 2011

42   *IARC handbooks of cancer prevention*, volume 8, fruits and vegetables. IARC Press. 2003 Page 12

43   Harbans L. Bhardwaj and Anwar A. Hamama Effect of Cultivar and Growing Location on the Mineral Composition of Canola Sprouts. HortScience. 2009

44   Touillaud MS, Thiébaut AC, Fournier A, et al. Dietary Lignan Intake and Post-menopausal Breast Cancer Risk by Estrogen and Progesterone Receptor Status. J Natl Cancer Inst. 2007

45   Wang XY, Nie GN, Yang HY et al. Chinese Medicine for menopausal syndrome: current status, problems and strategies. Chin J Integr Med. 2011

46   Currier, Andrew F. The Menopause: A Consideration of the Phenomena Which Occur to Women at the Close of the Child Bearing Period (1897)

47   Gengli Zhao, Linhong Wang, Renying Yan, et al. Menopausal symptoms: experience of Chinese women. Climacteric. 2000

48   Goldin BR, Adlercreutz H, Dwyer JT, et al. Effect of diet on excretion of estrogens in pre- and postmenopausal women. Cancer Res. 1981

49   Eric Hobsbawm, *The Age of Revolution: Europe 1789–1848*, Weidenfeld & Nicolson Ltd., p. 27. 1961

50   Yewoubdari Beyenene From menarche to menopause. State University New York. 1989

51   Ruiz-Núñez B, Pruimboom L, Dijck-Brouwer DA, et al. Lifestyle and nutritional imbalances associated with Western diseases: causes and consequences of chronic systemic low-grade inflammation in an evolutionary context. Jour Nutr Biochem. 2013

52   Prior JC, Naess M, Langhammer A, et al. Ovulation Prevalence in Women with Spontaneous Normal-Length Menstrual Cycles - A Population-Based Cohort from HUNT, Norway. PLOS One 2015

53   Zanetta GM, Webb MJ and Li H. Hyperestrogenism. A relevant risk factor for the development of cancer from endometriosis. Gynecologic Oncology. 2000

54   Bolton JL, Pisha E, Zhang F et al. Role of quinoids in estrogen carcinogenesis. (1998) Chem Res Toxicol. 1998

55   Tam IS and Giguère V. There and back again: The journey of the estrogen-related receptors in the cancer realm. J Steroid Biochem Mol Biol. 2016

56   Deroo BJ and Buensuceso AV.Minireview: Estrogen receptor-beta: mechanistic insights from recent studies. Mol Endocrinol. 2010

57   Thornton MJ. Estrogen functions in skin and skin appendages. Expert Opin Ther Targets. 2005

58   Jaisamrarn U, Triratanachat S, Chaikittisilpa S, et al. Ultra-low-dose estriol and lactobacilli in the local treatment of postmenopausal vaginal atrophy. Climacteric. 2013

59   Nikolaos Samaras, Maria-Aikaterini Papadopoulou and Dimitrios Samaras, et al. Off-label use of hormones as an antiaging strategy: a review Clin Interv Aging. 2014

60   Douglas C Hall. Nutritional Influences on Estrogen Metabolism. Nutri Advanced. 2001

61   Lee John, (with Victoria Hopkins) *What Your Doctor May Not Tell You About Menopause*. 1996 Warner Books. Page 163

62   Jarošová B, Erseková A, Hilscherová K, et al. Europe-wide survey of estrogenicity in wastewater treatment plant effluents: the need for the effect-based monitoring. Environ Sci Pollut Res Int. 2014

63   Carson, R. S*ilent Spring.* Abe Books. 1962

64   Diamanti-Kandarakis E, Bourguignon JP, Giudice LC, et al. Endocrine-disrupting chemicals: an Endocrine Society scientific statement. Endocr Rev. 2009

65   Craig ZR, Wang W and Flaws JA. Endocrine-disrupting chemicals in ovarian function: effects on steroidogenesis, metabolism and nuclear receptor signaling. Reproduction. 2011

66   Mlynarcikova A, Fickova M and Scsukova S. Impact of endocrine disruptors on ovarian steroidogenesis. Endocr Regul. 2014

67   Davey DA. HRT: some unresolved clinical issues in breast cancer, endometrial cancer and premature ovarian insufficiency. Womens Health (Lond). 2013

68   Mayor S. Continuous HRT with estrogen plus progestogen is linked to reduced risk of endometrial cancer. BMJ. 2015

69   Meendering JR, Torgrimson BN, Miller NP, et al. Estrogen, medroxyprogesterone acetate, endothelial function, and biomarkers of cardiovascular risk in young women. Am J Physiol Heart Circ. 2008

70   Li CI, Beaber EF, Tang MT, et al. Effect of depo-medroxyprogesterone acetate on breast cancer risk among women 20 to 44 years of age. Cancer Res. 2012

71   Birrell SN, Butler LM, Harris JM, et al. Disruption of androgen receptor signalling by synthetic progestins may increase risk of developing breast cancer. FASEB J. 2007

72   Lok Wong K, Ming Lai Y, Li KW, et al. A Novel, Stable, Estradiol-Stimulating, Osteogenic Yam Protein with Potential for the Treatment of Menopausal Syndrome. Sci Rep. 2015

73   Lee, J. (with Victoria Hopkins) *What your doctor may not tell you about menopause.* 1996 Little, Brown and Company. Page 167

74   Benster B, Carey A, Wadsworth F, et al. Double-blind placebo-controlled study to evaluate the effect of pro-juven progesterone cream on atherosclerosis and bone density. Menopause Int. 2009

75   Benster B, Carey A, Wadsworth F, et al. A double-blind placebo-controlled study to evaluate the effect of progestelle progesterone cream on postmenopausal women. (2009). Menopause Int. 2009

76   Zava DT, Dollbaum CM and Blen M. Estrogen and progestin bioactivity of foods, herbs, and spices. Proc Soc Exp Biol Med. 1998

77   Kuiper GG, Lemmen JG and Carlsson B. Interaction of estrogenic chemicals and phytoestriol estrogens with estrogen receptor β. Endocrinology. 1998

78   Deroo BJ and Buensuceso AV. Minireview: Estrogen receptor-beta: mechanistic insights from recent studies. Mol Endocrinol. 2010

79   Hughes C and Tansey G. Phytestrogens and Reproductive Medicine. The Reproductive and developmental toxicology. Ed. Corach KS Marcel Dekker Inc. New York 1998. Page 281

80   Kojima H, Takeda Y, Muromoto R, et al. Isoflavones enhance interleukin-17 gene expression via retinoic acid receptor-related orphan receptors α and γ. Toxicology. 2015

81   Mullican SE, DiSpirito JR, and Lazar MA. The Orphan Nuclear Receptors at Their 25th Year Reunion. J Mol Endocrinol. 2013

82   Komesaroff PA, Black CV, Cable V, et al. Effects of wild yam extract on menopausal symptoms, lipids and sex hormones in healthy menopausal women. Climacteric. 2001

83   Toh MF, Sohn J, Chen SN, et al. Biological characterization of non-steroidal progestins from botanicals used for women's health. Steroids. 2012

84   Toh MF, Mendonca E, Eddie SL, et al. Kaempferol Exhibits Progestogenic Effects in Ovariectomized Rats. J Steroids Horm Sci. 2014

85   Burdette, JE. And Murphy, B. Botanical derived progestins and their impact on women's health, (currently being undertaken at the University of Illinois at Chicago, Chicago, IL, United States).

86   Chen AY and Chen YC. A review of the dietary flavonoid, kaempferol on human health and cancer chemoprevention. Food Chem. 2014

87   Zhang Y, Chen AY, Li M, et al. Ginkgo biloba extract kaempferol inhibits cell proliferation and induces apoptosis in pancreatic cancer cells. J Surg Res. 2008

88   Hyun Sook Lee, Han Jin Cho, , et al. Mechanisms Underlying Apoptosis-Inducing Effects of Kaempferol in HT-29 Human Colon Cancer cells. Int J Mol Sci. 2014

89   Xie F, Su,M, Zhang QM, et al. Kaempferol Promotes Apoptosis in Human Bladder Cancer Cells by Inducing the Tumor Suppressor, PTEN. Int J Mol Sci. 2013

90   Haitao Luo, Bingbing, Jiang, Bingyun Li, et al. Kaempferol nanoparticles achieve strong and selective inhibition of ovarian cancer cell viability. Int J Nanomedicine. 2012

91   Mak P, Leung YK , Tang WY et al. Apigenin Suppresses Cancer Cell Growth through ERβ1. Neoplasia. 2006

92   Anicki BJ, Upcewicz BA, Apiera AN et al. Effect of Temperature and Light (UV, IR) on Flavonol Content in Radish and Alfalfa Sprouts. Folia Biologica 2005

93   Thompson LU, Boucher BA, Liu Z, Cotterchio M, et al. Phytestrogen content of foods consumed in Canada, including isoflavones, lignans, and coumestans. Nutr Cancer. 2006

94   Benayad Z, Gómez-Cordovés C and Es-Safi NE. Identification and quantification of flavonoid glycosides from fenugreek (Trigonella foenum-graecum) germinated seeds by LC-DAD-ESI/MS analysis. J Food Comp. 2014

95   Tucci M and Benghuzzi H. Structural changes in the kidney associated with ovariectomy and diosgenin replacement therapy in adult female rats. Biomed Sci Instrum. 2003

96   Hajirahimkhan A, Dietz BM and Bolton JL. Botanical Modulation of menopausal symptoms: Mechanisms of Action. Pharmacol Rev. 2016

97   Toh MF and Burdette JE. Identifying Botanical Mechanisms of Action. Fitoterapia. 2011

98   Egner PA, Chen JG, Zarth AT, et al. Rapid and sustainable detoxication of airborne pollutants by broccoli sprout beverage: results of a randomized clinical trial in China. Cancer Prev Res (Phila). 2014

99   Watson GW, Beaver LM, Williams DE, et al. Phytochemicals from Cruciferous Vegetables, Epigenetics, and Prostate Cancer Prevention. AAPS J. 2013

100 Tang L, Zhang Y, Jobson HE, Li J, et al. Potent activation of mitochondria-mediated apoptosis and arrest in S and M phases of cancer cells by a broccoli sprout extract. Mol Cancer Ther. 2006

101 Wang X, Di Pasqua AJ, Govind S, et al. Selective depletion of mutant p53 by cancer chemopreventive isothiocyanates and their structure-activity relationships. J Med Chem. 2011

102 Fahey JW, Zhang Y, and Talalay P. Broccoli sprouts: An exceptionally rich source of inducers of enzymes that protect against chemical carcinogens. Proc Natl Acad Sci U S A. 1997

103   Noah TL, Zhang H, Zhou H, et al. Effect of broccoli sprouts on nasal response to live attenuated influenza virus in smokers: a randomized, double-blind study. PLoS One. 2014

104   Fowke JH, Loncope C, and Herbert JR. Brassica Vegetable Consumption Shifts Estrogen Metabolism in Healthy Postmenopausal Women. Cancer Epidemiol Biomarkers Prev. 2000

105   Auborn KJ, Fan S, Rosen EM, Goodwin L, et al. Indole-3-carbinol is a negative regulator of estrogen. J Nutr. 2003

106   Lin H, Gao X, Chen G, et al. Indole-3-carbinol as inhibitors of glucocorticoid-induced apoptosis in osteoblastic cells through blocking ROS-mediated Nrf2 pathway. Biochem Biophys Res Commun. 2015

107   Perez-Chacon G, de Los Rios C and Zapata JM. Indole-3-carbinol induces cMYC and IAP-family downmodulation and promotes apoptosis of Epstein-Barr virus (EBV)-positive but not of EBV-negative Burkitt's lymphoma cell lines. Pharmacol Res. 2014

108   Aronchik I, Kundu A, Quirit JG and Firestone GL. The antiproliferative response of indole-3-carbinol in human melanoma cells is triggered by an interaction with NEDD4-1 and disruption of wild-type PTEN degradation. Mol Cancer Res. 2014

109   Kundu A, Quirit JG, Khouri MG, Firestone GL. Inhibition of oncogenic BRAF activity by indole-3-carbinol disrupts microphthalmia-associated transcription factor expression and arrests melanoma cell proliferation. Mol Carcinog. 2017

110   Bryson, Bill, *At Home.* Transworld Digital. 2010. p 130.

111   Wallig MA, Heinz-Taheny KM, Epps DL, et al. Synergy among phytochemicals within crucifers: does it translate into chemoprotection? J Nutr. 2005

112   Link, LB, Potter, JD. Raw versus cooked vegetables and cancer risk. Cancer Epidemiol. Biomarkers Prev. 2004

113   Shekib LA. Nutritional improvement of lentils, chick pea, rice and wheat by natural fermentation. Plant Foods Hum Nutr. 1994

114   Marton M, Mandolki, ZS, Csapo-Kiss ZS, et al. The role of sprouts in human nutrition. A review. Sapientia–Hungarian University of Transylvania. 2010

115   Franchthi Cave And The Beginning Of Settled Village Life In Greece. Thomas W. Jacobson. *www.ascsa.edu.gr/pdf/uploads/hesperia/147874.pdf*

116   Lampe JW, Karr SC, Hutchins AM et al. Urinary equol excretion with a soy challenge: influence of habitual diet. Proc Soc Exp Biol Med. 1998

117   Duh PD, Du PC and Yen GC. Action of methanolic extract of mung bean hulls as inhibitors of lipid peroxidation and non-lipid oxidative damage. Food Chem Toxicol. 1999

118   Herrick JW. Native American and menopausal use of red clover Iroquois medical botany. (dissertaton) University of New York. 1977

119   *Phytochemicals of Nutraceutical Importance* (2014) edited by Dhan Prakash, Girish Sharma. p 156

120 Gaweł E. Chemical composition of lucerne (alaflafa) leaf extract (EFL) and its applications as a phytobiotic in human nutrition. Acta Sci Pol Technol Aliment. 2012

121 McNaughton SA and Marks GC. Development of a food composition database for the estimation of dietary intakes of glucosinolates, the biologically active constituents of cruciferous vegetables. Br J Nutr. 2003

122 Amanda Rao, Elizabeth Steels, Gavin Beccaria, et al. Influence of a Specialized Trigonella foenum-graecum Seed Extract (Libifem), on Testosterone, Estradiol and Sexual Function in Healthy Menstruating Women, a Randomised Placebo Controlled Study. Phytother Res. 2015

123 Saleh Rayyan, Torgils Fossen and Øyvind M. Andersen. Flavone C-Glycosides from Seeds of Fenugreek, Trigonella foenum-graecum L. J Agric Food Chem. 2010

124 Sevil Hakimi, Sakineh Mohammad-Alizadeh, Siahi MR, et al. Effect of Fenugreek seed on early menopausal symptoms. Tabriz University of Medical Sciences. 2005

125 International Sprout Growers Association Data. *www.sproutnet.com/Mung-Bean-Sprouts*

126 Faber KA and Hughes CL. The effect of neonatal exposure to diethylstilbestrol, genistein, and zearalenone on pituitary responsiveness and sexually dimorphic nucleus volume in the castrated adult rat. Biol Reprod. 1991

127 Keay J and Thornton JW. Hormone-activated estrogen receptors in annelid invertebrates: implications for evolution and endocrine disruption. Endocrinology. 2009

128 Hughes C and Tansey G. Phytestrogens and Reproductive Medicine. The Reproductive and developmental toxicology. Ed. Corach KS. Marcel Dekker Inc. New York 1998. Page 295

129 Wasserman MD, Taylor-Gutt A, Jessica M. Rothman, et al. Estrogenic plant foods of red colobus monkeys and mountain gorillas in Uganda. Am J Phys Anthropol. 2012

130 Bown, SR. *The Age of Scurvy.*. Summersdale; 2nd New edition edition (1 Feb. 2004) Page 9

131 *Ibid*

132 Jeremy Hugh Baron, Sailors' scurvy before and after James Lind – a reassessment. 2009, a Review Vol 67 page 317.

133 Bown, SR. *The Age of Scurvy.* Summersdale; 2nd New edition edition (1 Feb. 2004) Page 11

134 Lind J. A Treastie of the Scurvy in Three Parts. Containing an Inquiry into the Nature, Causes and Cure of that Disease, together with a critical and Chronological View of what has been published on the subject. Edinburgh. 1753

135 Maxwell, John. C. *Maxewell's 2 in 1.Developing the leader within you. Developing the leaders around you.* 2000. Thomas Nelson. p P55

136 Royal Geographical Society. *Explorers: Tales of Endurance and Exploration.* DK Publishing. 2010

137 Brandt, Anthony. *The Man Who Ate His Boots: Sir John Franklin and the Tragic History of the North West Passage.* Jonathan Cape. 2011 p 154

138 Wessley, John. *Primitive Physic, an easy and natural way of curing most diseases.* Initially published anonymously in 1747 but he reverted to his own name in 1791

139 Bown, SR. *The Age of Scurvy..* Summersdale; 2nd New edition edition (1 Feb. 2004) p 102

140 Tickner FJ and Medvei VC. Scurvy and the health or European crews in the Indian Ocean in the seventeenth century. Med History. 1958

141 Sir Thomas Browne's Works: Pseudodoxia epidemica, books 4-7. The garden of Cyrus. 1835 William Pickering (London) Page 435

142 Chung TY, Nwokolo EN, and Sim JS. Compositional and digestibility changes in sprouted barley and canola seeds. Plant Foods Hum Nutr. 1989

143 Bown, SR. *The Age of Scurvy.* Summersdale; 2nd New edition edition (1 Feb. 2004) Page 220

144 Y Nakamua, S Tsuji, and Y Tonogal. Determination of the levels of isoflavonoids in soybeans and soy derived foods and estimation of isoflavonoids in the Japanese daily intake. J AOAC Int. 2000

145 de Kleijn MJ, van der Schouw YT, Wilson PW, et al. Intake of dietary phytestrogens is low in postmenopausal women in the United States: the Framingham study(1-4). J Nutr. 2001. NOTE This study calculated in micrograms (ugs) which I have converted to milligrams (mgs).

146 Touillaud MS, Thiébaut AC, Fournier A, et al. Dietary lignan intake and postmenopausal breast cancer risk by estrogen and progesterone receptor status. J Natl Cancer Inst. 2007

147 Bhakta D, dos Santos Silva I, Higgins C, et al. A semiquantitative food frequency questionnaire is a valid indicator of the usual intake of phytestrogens by south Asian women in the UK relative to multiple 24-h dietary recalls and multiple plasma samples. J Nutr. 2005

148   Hedelin M, Löf M, Olsson M, et al. Dietary phytestrogens are not associated with risk of overall breast cancer but diets rich in coumestrol are inversely associated with risk of estrogen receptor and progesterone receptor negative breast tumors in Swedish women. J Nutr. 2008

149 J Surh, MJ Kim E Koh and Kim H Kwon. Estimates intakes of isoflaovnes and coumestrol in Korean population. Int J Food Sci Nutr. 2006

150 Boué SM, Wiese TE, Nehls S, et al. Evaluation of the estrogenic effects of legume extracts containing phytestrogens. J Agric Food Chem. 2003

151 Lampe JW, Karr SC, Hutchins AM, et al. Urinary equol excretion with a soy challenge: influence of habitual diet. Proc Soc Exp Biol Med. 1998

152 Adlercreutz, H. Human Health and Phytestrogens. Korach KS Ed. Reproductive and Developmental Toxicology. Marcel Dekker Inc. New York 1998 p 321

153 Bowe J, Li XF, Sugden D, Katzenellenbogen JA, et al. The effects of the phytestrogen, coumestrol, on gonadotropin-releasing hormone (GnRH) mRNA expression in GT1-7 GnRH neurones. J Neuroendocrinol. 2003

154 Cetisli NE, Saruhan A, Kivcak B. The effects of flaxseed on menopausal symptoms and quality of life. Holist Nurs Pract. 2015

155 Lee, J. (with Hopkins V) *What your doctor may not tell you about menopause.* Little, Brown and Company. 1996. Page 122

156 Hueston CM and Deak T. On the time course, generality, and regulation of plasma progesterone release in male rats by stress exposure. Endocrinology. 2014

157 Rimoldi G, Christoffel J, Seidlova-Wuttke D, et al. Effects of chronic genistein treatment in mammary gland, uterus, and vagina. W. Environ Health Perspect. 2007

158 Caruso S, Cianci S, Amore FF, et al. Quality of life and sexual function of naturally postmenopausal women on an ultralow-concentration estriol vaginal gel. Menopause. 2016

159 Krause M, Thomas L. Wheeler, II, et al. Local Effects of Vaginally Administered Estrogen Therapy: A Review Cochrane Database Syst Rev. 2009

160 Adlercreutz H, Mousavi Y, Clark J, et al. Dietary phytestrogens and cancer: in vitro and in vivo studies. Steroid Biochem Mol Biol. 1992

161 Nowak DA, Snyder DC, Brown AJ, et al. The Effect of Flaxseed Supplementation on Hormonal Levels Associated with Polycystic Ovarian Syndrome: A Case Study. Curr Top Nutraceutical Res. 2007

162 Monroe KR, Murphy SP, Henderson BE, et al. Dietary fiber intake and endogenous serum hormone levels in naturally postmenopausal Mexican American women: the Multiethnic Cohort Study. Nutr Cancer. 2007

163 Çakir E, Topaloğlu O, Çolak Bozkurt N, et al. Insulin-like growth factor 1, liver enzymes, and insulin resistance in patients with PCOS and hirsutism. Turk J Med Sci. 2014

164 Bühler-Christen A, Tischler V, Diener PA, et al. New onset alopecia and hirsutism in a postmenopausal women. Gynecol Endocrinol 2009

165 Fooladi E, Bell RJ, Jane F, et al. Testosterone improves antidepressant-emergent loss of libido in women: findings from a randomized, double-blind, placebo-controlled trial. J Sex Med. 2014

166 Reed BG, Bou Nemer L and Carr BR. Has testosterone passed the test in premenopausal women with low libido? A systematic review. Int J Womens Health. 2016

167 Rao A, Steels E, Beccaria G, et al. Influence of a Specialized Trigonella foenum-graecum Seed Extract (Libifem), on Testosterone, Estradiol and Sexual Function in Healthy Menstruating Women, a Randomised Placebo Controlled Study. Phytother Res. 2015

168 Rao A, Steels E, Inder WJ, et al. Testofen, a specialised Trigonella foenum-graecum seed extract reduces age-related symptoms of androgen decrease, increases testos-

terone levels and improves sexual function in healthy aging males in a double-blind randomised clinical study. Aging Male. 2016

169 Sato K, Fujita S and Iemitsu M. Acute administration of diosgenin or dioscorea improves hyperglycemia with increases muscular steroidogenesis in STZ-induced type 1 diabetic rats. J Steroid Biochem Mol Biol. 2014

170 Spandan Chaudhary, Surendra K. Chikara, Mahesh C. Sharma, et al. Elicitation of Diosgenin Production in Trigonella foenum-graecum (Fenugreek) Seedlings by Methyl Jasmonate. Int J Mol Sci. 2015

171 Styrczewska M, Kulma A, Kostyn K, et al. Flax terpenoid pathway as a source of health promoting compounds. Mini Rev Med Chem. 2013.

172 Shah SM, Ali S, Zubair M, et al. Effect of supplementation of feed with Flaxseed (Linumusitatisimum) oil on libido and semen quality of Nilli-Ravi buffalo bulls. J Anim Sci Technol. 2016

173 DeLamater J, Hyde JS and Fong MC. Sexual satisfaction in the seventh decade of life. J Sex Marital Ther. 2008

174 Stephanie M. Tortorella, Simon G. Royce, Paul V. Licciardi, et al. Dietary Sulforaphane in Cancer Chemoprevention: The Role of Epigenetic Regulation and HDAC Inhibition. Antioxid Redox Signal. 2015.

175 T A Shapiro, J W Fahey, K L Wade, et al. Human metabolism and excretion of cancer chemoprotective glucosinolates and isothiocyanates of cruciferous vegetables. Cancer Epidemiol Biomarkers Prev. 1998

176 Rajendran P, Dashwood WM, Li L, Kang et al. Nrf2 status affects tumor growth, HDAC3 gene promoter associations, and the response to sulforaphane in the colon. Clin Epigenetics. 2015

177 Liu CM, Peng CY, Liao YW, et al. Sulforaphane targets cancer stemness and tumor initiating properties in oral squamous cell carcinomas via miR-200c induction. Journal of the Formosan Medical Association. 2016

178 Omkara L. Veeranki, Arup Bhattacharya, et al. Organ-specific exposure and response to sulforaphane, a key chemopreventive ingredient in broccoli: implications for cancer prevention. Br J Nutr. 2013

179 Brian S. Cornblatt Lingxiang Ye, Albena T, et al. Preclinical and clinical evaluation of sulforaphane for chemoprevention in the breast. Carcinogenesis 2007

180 Clarke JD, Riedl K, Bella D, et al. Comparison of isothiocyanate metabolite levels and histone deacetylase activity in human subjects consuming broccoli sprouts or broccoli supplement. J Agric Food Chem. 2011

181 Clarke JD, Hsu A, Riedl K, Bella D, et al. Bioavailability and inter-conversion of sulforaphane and erucin in human consuming broccoli sprouts or broccoli supplement in a cross-over study design. Pharmacol Res. 2011

182 *www.dailymail.co.uk/health/article-3343559/How-broccoli-help-fight-CANCER-Compound-halts-growth-colon-prostate-cancer-cells-makes-treatment-effective.html*

183   Xu L, Cao J and Chen W. Structural characterization of a broccoli polysaccharide and evaluation of anti-cancer cell proliferation effects. Carbohydr Polym. 2015

184   Bosetti C, Filomeno M, Riso P, et al. Cruciferous vegetables and cancer risk in a network of case-control studies. Ann Oncol. 2012

185   Myzak MC, Tong P, Dashwood WM, et al. Sulforaphane retards the growth of human PC-3 xenografts and inhibits HDAC activity in human subjects. Exp Biol Med (Maywood). 2007

186   Mandeep K. Virk-Baker, Tim R. Nagy, et al. Role of phytestrogens in cancer therapy. Planta Med. 2010

187   Paige E. Miller and Denise C. Snyder. Phytochemicals and cancer risk: a review of the epidemiological evidence. Nutr Clin Pract. 2012

188   Velentzis LS, Cantwell MM, Cardwell C, et al. Lignans and breast cancer risk in pre- and post-menopausal women: meta-analyses of observational studies. Br J Cancer. 2009

189   Tham DM, Gardner CD, and Haskell WL. Potential Health Benefits of Dietary Phytestrogens: A Review of the Clinical, Epidemiological, and Mechanistic Evidence. J Clin Endocrinol Metab. 1998

190   Thompson LU, Chen JM and Li T. Dietary flaxseed alters tumor biological markers in postmenopausal breast cancer. Clin Cancer Res. 2005.

191   Lee J and Cho K. Flaxseed sprouts induce apoptosis and inhibit growth in MCF-7 and MDA-MB-231 human breast cancer cells. In Vitro Cell Dev Biol Anim. 2012

192   Buck K, Zaineddin AK, Vrieling A, et al. Estimated enterolignans, lignan-rich foods, and fibre in relation to survival after postmenopausal breast cancer. Br J Cancer. 2011

193   *www.oncologynutrition.org/erfc/hot-topics/flaxseeds-and-breast-cancer*

194   Raju KS, Taneja I, Valicherla GR, et al. No effect on pharmacokinetics of tamoxifen and 4-hydroxytamoxifen by multiple doses of red clover capsule in rats. Sci Rep. 2015

195   Chen J, Hui E, Ip T, et al. Dietary flaxseed enhances the inhibitory effect of tamoxifen on the growth of estrogen-dependent human breast cancer (mcf-7) in nude mice. Clin Cancer Res. 2004

196   Chen J, Power KA, Mann J, et al. Flaxseed alone or in combination with tamoxifen inhibits MCF-7 breast tumor growth in ovariectomized athymic mice with high circulating levels of estrogen. Exp Biol Med (Maywood). 2007

197   McCann SE, Edge SB, Hicks DG, et al. A Pilot Study Comparing the Effect of Flaxseed, Aromatase Inhibitor, and the Combination on Breast Tumor Biomarkers. Nutr Cancer. 2014

198   Lephart ED. Review Article Modulation of Aromatase by Phytestrogens. Enzyme Res. 2015

199   Shin S, Saito E, Inoue M, et al. Dietary pattern and breast cancer risk in Japanese women: the Japan Public Health Center-based Prospective Study. JPHC Study 2016

200 Weaver CM, Alekel L, Ward WE, et al. Flavonoid Intake and Bone Health. J Nutr Gerontol Geriatr. 2012

201 Setchell KD and Lydeking-Olsen E. Dietary phytestrogens and their effect on bone: evidence from in vitro and in vivo, human observational, and dietary intervention studies. Am J Clin Nutr. 2003

202 Cegieła U, Folwarczna J, Pytlik M, et al. Effects of Extracts from Trifolium medium L. and Trifolium pratense L. on Development of Estrogen Deficiency-Induced Osteoporosis in Rats. Evid Based Complement Alternat Med. 2012

203 Occhiuto F, Pasquale RD, Guglielmo G, et al. Effects of phytestrogenic isoflavones from red clover (Trifolium pratense L.) on experimental osteoporosis. Phytother Res. 2007

204 Kawakita S, Marotta F, Naito Y, et al. Effect of an isoflavones-containing red clover preparation and alkaline supplementation on bone metabolism in ovariectomized rats. Clin Interv Aging. 2009

205 Kaczmarczyk-Sedlak I, Wojnar W, Zych M, et al. Effect of formononetin on mechanical properties and chemical composition of bones in rats with ovariectomy-induced osteoporosis. Evid Based Complement Alternat Med. 2013

206 Thorup AC, Lambert MN, Strøm Kahr H et al. Intake of Novel Red Clover Supplementation for 12 Weeks Improves Bone Status in Healthy Menopausal Women. Evid Based Complement Alternat Med. 2015

207 Yang L, Takai H, Utsunomiya T, et al. Kaempferol stimulates bone sialoprotein gene transcription and new bone formation. J Cell Biochem. 2010.

208 Goto T, Hagiwara K, Shirai N, et al. Apigenin inhibits osteoblastogenesis and osteoclastogenesis and prevents bone loss in ovariectomized mice. Cytotechnology. 2015

209 Horcajada MN and Offord E. Naturally plant-derived compounds: role in bone anabolism. Curr Mol Pharmacol. 2012

210 Juma Ab. The effects of Lepidium sativum seeds on fracture-induced healing in rabbits. MedGenMed. 2007

211 Raval ND and Pandya TN. Clinical trial of Lepidium Sativum Linn(Chandrashura) in the management of Sandhivata(Osteoarthritis). Jamnagar. Ayu. 2009

212 Shanb AA andYoussef EF. The impact of adding weight-bearing exercise versus nonweight bearing programs to the medical treatment of elderly patients with osteoporosis. J Family Community Med. 2014

213 Ha V, Sievenpiper JL, de Souza RJ, et al. Effect of dietary pulse intake on established therapeutic lipid targets for cardiovascular risk reduction: a systematic review and meta-analysis of randomized controlled trials. CMAJ. 2014

214 Sato S, Mukai Y, Yamate J, Kato J, et al. Effect of polyphenol-containing azuki bean (Vigna angularis) extract on blood pressure elevation and macrophage infiltration in the heart and kidney of spontaneously hypertensive rats. Clin Exp Pharmacol Physiol. 2008

215   Kim M, Kim DK and Cha YS. Black Adzuki Bean (Vigna angularis) Extract
       Protects Pancreatic β Cells and Improves Glucose Tolerance in C57BL/6J Mice Fed
       a High-Fat Diet. J Med Food. 2016

216   Kim M, Park JE, Song SB, et al. Effects of black adzuki bean (Vigna angularis)
       extract on proliferation and differentiation of 3T3-L1 preadipocytes into mature
       adipocytes. Nutrients. 2015

217   Kitano-Okada T, Ito A, Koide A, et al. Anti-obesity role of adzuki bean extract
       containing polyphenols: in vivo and in vitro effects. J Sci Food Agric. 2012

218   Tang D, Dong Y, Ren H, et al A review of phytochemistry, metabolite changes,
       and medicinal uses of the common food mung bean and its sprouts (Vigna radiata).
       Chem Cent J. 2014

219   Winham DM and Hutchins AM. Perceptions of flatulence from bean consumption
       among adults in 3 feeding studies. Nutr J. 2011

220   Peñalvo JL and López-Romero P. Urinary enterolignan concentrations are positive-
       ly associated with serum HDL cholesterol and negatively associated with serum
       triglycerides in U.S. adults. J Nutr. 2012

221   Bosely Sarah. A Million Women can't be wrong The Guardian. Monday 16 March
       2009

222   "HRT And The Menopause - Live Well - NHS Choices". *www.nhs.uk/Livewell/*
       menopause/Pages/HormoneReplacementTherapy.aspx

223   Gigi Engle. "The Science Of Better Sex: Why Orgasms Only Get Better With Age".
       Elite Daily. *www.elitedaily.com/dating/it-all-gets-better-with-age/906428/*

224   Steels E, Rao A, and Vitetta L. Physiological Aspects of Male Libido Enhanced
       by Standardized Trigonella foenum-graecum Extract and Mineral Formulation.
       Phytother Res. 2011

225   Trompeter SE, Bettencourt R, and Barrett-Connor E. Sexual Activity and Satisfac-
       tion in Healthy Community-dwelling Older Women. Am J Med. 2012

226   Deborah Giles, speaking on BBC Radion 4 Program "The Whale Menopause"
       First aired 10th August 2016

227   Marchesi JR, Adams DH, Fava F, et al. The gut microbiota and host health: a new
       clinical frontier. Gut. 2016

228   Fredua-Agyeman M and Gaisford S. Comparative survival of commercial probiotic
       formulations: tests in biorelevant gastric fluids and real-time measurements using
       microcalorimetry. Benef Microbes. 2015

229   Selma MV, Espín JC and Tomás-Barberán FA. Interaction between phenolics and
       gut microbiota: role in human health. J Agric Food Chem. 2009

230   Tugba Ozdal , David A. Sela , Jianbo Xiao, et al. The Reciprocal Interactions be-
       tween Polyphenols and Gut Microbiota and Effects on Bioaccessibility. Nutrients.
       2016

231   Burow M, Bergner A, Gershenzon J et al. Glucosinolate hydrolysis in Lepidium
       sativum--identification of the thiocyanate-forming protein. Plant Mol Biol. 2007

232 Durham P and Poulton JE. Effect of Castanospermine and Related Polyhydroxy-alkaloids on Purified Myrosinase from Lepidium sativum Seedlings. Plant Physiol. 1989

233 Clarke JD, Hsu A, Riedl K et al. Bioavailability and inter-conversion of sulfora-phane and erucin in human subjects consuming broccoli sprouts or broccoli supplement in a cross-over study design. Pharmacol Res. 2011

234 Cramer JM, Jeffery EH. Sulforaphane absorption and excretion following ingestion of a semi-purified broccoli powder rich in glucoraphanin and broccoli sprouts in healthy men. Nutr Cancer. 2011

235 Angelino D, Dosz EB, Sun J et al. Myrosinase-dependent and -independent formation and control of isothiocyanate products of glucosinolate hydrolysis. Front Plant Sci. 2015

236 Tworoger ST, Rosner BA, Willett WC, et al. The combined influence of multiple sex and growth hormones on risk of postmenopausal breast cancer: a nested case-control study. Breast Cancer Res. 2011

237 The liver's role in hormone balance. The Educational Resource Centre of the Women's International Pharmacy. 2011 *www.womensinternational.com/connections/liver/*

238 Klontz KC, DeBeck HJ, LeBlanc P, et al. The Role of Adverse Event Reporting in the FDA Response to a Multistate Outbreak of Liver Disease Associated with a Dietary Supplement. Public Health Rep. 2015

239 Bunchorntavakul C and Reddy KR. Review article: herbal and dietary supplement hepatotoxicity. Aliment Pharmacol Ther. 2013

240 Hfaiedh M, Brahmi D and Zourgui L. Hepatoprotective effect of Taraxacum officinale leaf extract on sodium dichromate-induced liver injury in rats. Environ Toxicol. 2016

241 Temple, N.J, Burkitt D.P (Eds) *Western Diseases: Their Dietary Prevention and Reversibility*. Humana Press. page 209 - 235

242 Temple VJ, Ighogboja IS and Okonji MC. Serum vitamin A and beta-carotene levels in pre-school age children. J Trop Pediatr. 1994

243 Michel T, Halabalaki M and Skaltsounis AL. New Concepts, Experimental Approaches, and Dereplication Strategies for the Discovery of Novel Phytestrogens from Natural Sources. Planta Med. 2013

244 Coulman KF and Cole SJ. Whole sesame seed is as rich a source of mammalian lignan precursors as whole flaxseed. Nutr Cancer. 2005

245 Boam T. Anti-androgenic effects of flavonols in prostate cancer. Ecancermedical-science. 2015

246 Maffini MV, Rubin BS, Sonnenschein C, et al. Endocrine disruptors and reproduc-tive health: the case of bisphenol-A. Mol Cell Endocrinol. 2006

247 Ziv-Gal A, and Flaws JA. Evidence for bisphenol A-induced female infertility: a review. Fertil Steril. 2016

248 Natalia M. Grindler, Jenifer E. Allsworth, et al. Persistent Organic Pollutants and Early Menopause in U.S. Women. PLoS One. 2015.

249 Darbre PD, Aljarrah A, Miller WR, et al. Concentrations of parabens in human breast tumours. J Appl Toxicol. 2004

250 Pan S, Yuan C, Tagmount A, et al. Parabens and human epidermal growth factor receptor ligand cross-talk in breast cancer cells. Environ Health Perspect. 2016

251 Lillo MA, Nichols C, Perry C Runke S, et al. Methylparaben stimulates tumor initiating cells in ER+ breast cancer models. J Appl Toxicol. 2017

252 Glenville M. *Natural Solutions to Menopause.* Rodale 2013 Kindle Edition Loc 1520

253 "Do Simple products contain Parabens." *www.simple.co.uk/about-us/ frequently-asked-questions/answer-detail/383343/*

254 Prest EI, Hammes F, van Loosdrecht MC, et al. Biological Stability of Drinking Water: Controlling Factors, Methods, and Challenges. Front Microbiol. 2016

255 Lipphaus P, Hammes F, Kötzsch S, et al. Microbiological tap water profile of a medium-sized building and effect of water stagnation. Environmental Technology. 2014

256 UK Environment Agency "Causes and consequences of feminisation of male fish in English rivers." *www.gov.uk/government/publications/causes-and-consequences-of-feminisation-of-male-fish-in-english-rivers* First published:1 July 2004

257 Skakkebaek NE, De Meyts ER, Buck Louis GM, et al. Male Reproductive Disorders and Fertility Trends: Influences of Environment and Genetic Susceptibility. Physiol Rev. 2016

258 Aravindakshan J, Gregory M, Marcogliese DJ, et al. Consumption of xenestrogen-contaminated fish during lactation alters adult male reproductive function. Toxicol Sci. 2004

259 These American Meat Products Are Banned Abroad by The Daily Meal. See *www.huffingtonpost.com/the-daily-meal/these-american-meat-produ_b_5153275.html* Updated Jun 16, 2014

260 Carwile JL, Willett WC, Spiegelman D, et al. Sugar-sweetened beverage consumption and age at menarche in a prospective study of US girls. Hum Reprod. 2015

261 Milton K. Micronutrient intakes of wild primates: are humans different? Comp Biochem Physiol A Mol Integr Physiol. 2003

262 Milton K, Jenness R. Ascorbic acid content of neotropical plant parts available to wild monkeys and bats. Experientia. 1987

263 Kim HY, Kim OH and Sung MK. Effects of phenol-depleted and phenol-rich diets on blood markers of oxidative stress, and urinary excretion of quercetin and kaempferol in healthy volunteers. J Am Coll Nutr. 2003

264 Vasconcelos AR, Yshii LM, Viel TA, et al. Intermittent fasting attenuates lipopolysaccharide-induced neuroinflammation and memory impairment. J Neuroinflammation. 2014

265 Vasconcelos AR, Kinoshita PF, Yshii LM, et al. Effects of intermittent fasting on age-related changes on Na,K-ATPase activity and oxidative status induced by lipopolysaccharide in rat hippocampus. Neurobiol Aging. 2015

266 Ghawi SK, Shen Y, Niranjan K, et al. Consumer acceptability and sensory profile of cooked broccoli with mustard seeds added to improve chemoprotective properties. J Food Sci. 2014

267 Ghawi SK, Methven L, and Niranjan K. The potential to intensify sulforaphane formation in cooked broccoli (Brassica oleracea var. italica) using mustard seeds (Sinapis alba). Food Chem. 2013.

268 Rovenský J, Stancíková M, Masaryk P, et al. Eggshell calcium in the prevention and treatment of osteoporosis. Int J Clin Pharmacol Res. 2003

269 Mony B, Ebenezar AV, Ghani MF, et al. Effect of Chicken Egg Shell Powder Solution on Early Enamel Carious Lesions: An Invitro Preliminary Study. J Clin Diagn Res. 2015

270 Rovenský J, Stancíková M, Masaryk P, et al. Eggshell calcium in the prevention and treatment of osteoporosis. Int J Clin Pharmacol Res. 2003

271 Masuda Y. Hen's eggshell calcium. Clin Calcium. 2005

272 Munch R and Barringer SA. Deodorization of garlic breath volatiles by food and food components. J Food Sci. 2014

273 Ragusa L, Picchi V, Tribulato A, et al. The effect of the germination temperature on the phytochemical content of broccoli and rocket sprouts. Int J Food Sci Nutr. 2017

274 Sangronis E and Machado CJ. Influence of germination on the nutritional quality of Phaseolus vulgaris and Cajanus cajan. LWT - Food Sci and Tech. 2005

275 Torsten Bohn. Dietary Factors Influencing Magnesium Absorption in Humans. Cur Nut & Food Sci. 2008

276 Reinhold JG, Nasr K, Lahimgarzadeh A, et al. Effects of purified phytate and phytate-rich bread upon metabolism of zinc, calcium, phosphorus, and nitrogen in man. Lancet 1973

277 Heaney RP, Weaver CM and Fitzsimmons ML. Soybean phytate content: effect on calcium absorption. Am J Clin Nutr. 1991

278 Campas-Baypoli ON, González-Pacheco E, Cantúsoto EU et al. Phenolic profile, antioxidant capacity and sulforaphane content during the storage of broccoli sprouts. Int J Pharma Bio Sci. 2014

279 Miglio C, Chiavaro E, Visconti A, et al. Effects of Different Cooking Methods on Nutritional and Physicochemical Characteristics of Selected Vegetables. J. Agric. Food Chem. 2008

280 Gao-feng Yuan, Bo Sun, Jing Yuan, et al. Effects of different cooking methods on health-promoting compounds of broccoli. Univ. Sci. B. 2009

281 Qiaoying Lv, Yi Yang, Yongxin Zhao, et al Comparative Study on Separation and Purification of Isoflavones from the Seeds and Sprouts of Chickpea by HSCCC. J Liq Chromatogr Relat Technol. 2009

282   Shuhui Zhao, Linping Zhang, Peng Gao, et al. Isolation and characterisation of the isoflavones from sprouted chickpea seeds. Food Chem 2009

283   Hai-rong Ma, Jie Wang, Hong-xue Qi, et al. Assessment of the estrogenic activities of chickpea (Cicer arietinum L) sprout isoflavone extract in ovariectomized rats. Acta Pharmacol Sin. 2013

284   Messina V. Nutritional and health benefits of dried beans. AJ Clin Nut. 2014

285   Dongyan T, Yinmao D, Li L, et al. Antioxidant activity in mung bean sprouts and safety of extracts for cosmetic use. J Cosmet Sci. 2014

286   Reena Randhir, Yuan-Tong Lin, Kalidas Shetty Stimulation of phenolics, antioxidant and antimicrobial activities in dark germinated mung bean sprouts in response to peptide and phytochemical elicitors. Pro Bio. 2004

287   Guo X, Li T, Tang K, et al. Effect of germination on phytochemical profiles and antioxidant activity of mung bean sprouts (Vigna radiata). J Agric Food Chem. 2012

288   Soucek J, Skvor J, Poucková P, et al. Mung bean sprout (Phaseolus aureus) nuclease and its biological and antitumor effects. Neoplasma. 2006

289   Yao Y, Chen F, Wang M, et al. Antidiabetic activity of Mung bean extracts in diabetic KK-Ay mice. J Agric Food Chem. 2008

290   Michał Świeca and Barbara Baraniak. Influence of elicitation with H2O2 on phenolics content, antioxidant potential and nutritional quality of Lens culinaris sprouts. J Sci Food Agric. 2014

291   Świeca M, Gawlik-Dziki U, Kowalczyk D, et al. Impact of germination time and type of illumination on the antioxidant compounds and antioxidant capacity of Lens culinaris sprouts. Sci Hort. 2012

292   Kanti Bhooshan Pandey and Syed Ibrahim Rizvi. Plant polyphenols as dietary antioxidants in human health and disease. Oxid Med Cell Longev. 2009

293   Yang Yao and Guixing Ren. Suppressive effect of extruded adzuki beans (Vigna angularis) on hyperglycemia after sucrose loading in rats. Ind Crop & Prod. 2013

294   Yang Yao, Xuzhen Chenga and Guixing Ren. α-Glucosidase inhibitory activity of protein-rich extracts from extruded adzuki bean in diabetic KK-Ay mice. Food & Function. 2014

295   White PJ and Broadley MR. Biofortification of crops with seven mineral elements often lacking in human diets--iron, zinc, copper, calcium, magnesium, selenium and iodine. New Phytol. 2009

296   Baumgart DC and Carding SR. Inflammatory bowel disease: cause and immunobiology. Lancet. 2007

297   Alves DL, Lima SM, da Silva CR, et al. Effects of Trifolium pratense and Cimicifuga racemosa on the endometrium of Wistar rats. Maturitas. 2008

298   USDA Database for the Flavonoid Content of Selected Foods. Release 3.1 Prepared May 2014 by Seema Bhagwat, David B. Haytowitz, and Joanne M. Holden

299 ChungJa J, VasanthaRupasinghe H. Tables of Isoflavone, Coumestan and Lignan Data. Phytestrogens and health ed. Edited by Anderson J.J.B Sarwar Gilani G. AOCS Publishing. 2002

300 Story JA, LePage SL, Petro MS, et al. Interactions of alfalfa plant and sprout saponins with cholesterol in vitro and in cholesterol-fed rats. Am J Clin Nutr. 1984

301 Malinow MR, McLaughlin P, Papworth L, et al. Effect of alfalfa saponins on intestinal cholesterol absorption in rats. Am J Clin Nutr. 1977

302 Rink, LD. Folic Acid and Alfalfa The Fall Study. Indiana University School of Medicine. 2003

303 Hong YH, Huang CJ, Wang SC, et al. The ethyl acetate extract of alfalfa sprout ameliorates disease severity of autoimmune-prone MRL-lpr/lpr mice. Lupus. 2009

304 Hong YH, Chao WW, Chen ML, et al. Ethyl acetate extracts of alfalfa (Medicago sativa L.) sprouts inhibit lipopolysaccharide-induced inflammation in vitro and in vivo. J Biomed Sci. 2009

305 Mirzaei A, Delaviz H, Mirzaei M, et al. The Effects of Medicago Sativa and Allium Porrum on Iron Overload in Rats. Glob J Health Sci. 2015

306 Tahany A. Aly S, Fayed, A et al Effect of Egyptian Radish and Clover Sprouts on Blood Sugar and Lipid Metabolisms in Diabetic Rats. Global J Biotech & Biochemi. 2015

307 Longxin Q, Tong Chen, Fojin Zhong et al. Red clover extract antidiabetic and hypolipidemic effects in db/db mice. Exp Ther Med 2014

308 Biljana K, Popovic M, Vlaisavljevic S et al. Antioxidant Profile of Trifolium pratense L. Molecules. 2012

309   Singh D, Connors SL, Macklin EA, et al. Sulforaphane treatment of autism spectrum disorder (ASD). Proc Natl Acad Sci U S A. 2014

310 Shiina A, Kanahara N, Sasaki T, et al. An Open Study of Sulforaphane-rich Brocco-li Sprout Extract in Patients with Schizophrenia. Clin Psychopharmacol Neurosci. 2015

311 Vasanthi HR, Mukherjee S, Das DK. Potential health benefits of broccoli- a chemico-biological overview. Mini Rev Med Chem. 2009

312 Bahadoran Z, Mirmiran P, Hosseinpanah F et al. Broccoli sprouts reduce oxidative stress in type 2 diabetes: a randomized double-blind clinical trial. Eur J Clin Nutr. 2011

313 Hanlon PR and Barnes DM. Phytochemical composition and biological activity of 8 varieties of radish (Raphanus sativus L.) sprouts and mature taproots. J Food Sci. 2011

314 Beevi SS, Mangamoori LN, Subathra M, et al. Hexane extract of Raphanus sativus L. roots inhibits cell proliferation and induces apoptosis in human cancer cells by modulating genes related to apoptotic pathway. Plant Foods Hum Nutr. 2010

315 O'Hare TJ, Williams DJ, Zhang B et al. Radish Sprouts Versus Broccoli Sprouts: A Comparison Of Anti-Cancer Potential Based On Glucosinolate Breakdown Products. ActaHortic. 2009

316 Taniguchi H, Kobayashi-Hattori K, Tenmyo C, et al. Effect of Japanese radish (Raphanus sativus) sprout (Kaiware-daikon) on carbohydrate and lipid metabolisms in normal and streptozotocin-induced diabetic rats. Phytother Res. 2006

317 Vivarelli F, Canistro D, Sapone A, et al. Raphanus sativus cv. Sango Sprout Juice Decreases Diet-Induced Obesity in Sprague Dawley Rats and Ameliorates Related Disorders. PLoS One. 2016

318 Baenas N, Piegholdt S, Schloesser A, et al. Metabolic Activity of Radish Sprouts Derived Isothiocyanates in Drosophila melanogaster. Int J Mol Sci. 2016

319 Mazur W. Phytestrogen content in foods. Baillieres Clin Endocrinol Metab. 1998

320 Haytowitz DB, Holden JM and Bhagwat S. USDA Database for the Isoflavone Content of Selected Foods Release 2.0 (2008)

321 Brooks JD, Ward WE, Lewis JE, et al. Supplementation with flaxseed alters estrogen metabolism in postmenopausal women to a greater extent than does supplementation with an equal amount of soy. Am J Clin Nutr. 2004

322 Żuk M, Kulma A, Dymińska L, et al. Flavonoid engineering of flax potentiate its biotechnological application. BMC Biotechnol. 2011

323 HPLC analysis of trigonella foenum-graecum seeds to assess phytestrogens. Int J Food Nutri Sci. 2014

324 Han Y, Nishibe S, Noguchi Y, et al. Flavonol glycosides from the stems of Trigonella foenum-graecum. Phytochemistry. 2001

325 Sreeja S, Anju VS and Sreeja S. In vitro estrogenic activities of fenugreek Trigonella foenum graecum seeds. Indian J Med Res. 2010

326 Djerassi C, Rosenkranz G, Pataki J, et al. Sterioids synthesis of allopregnane-3beta, 11beta, 17alpha-, 20beta, 21-pentol from cortisone and diosgenin. J Biol Chem. 1952

327 Chadha RK, Lawrence JF and Ratnayake WM. Ion chromatographic determination of cyanide released from flaxseed under autohydrolysis conditions. Food Addit Contam. 1995

328 Villeneuve S, Mondor M and Tsao R. Effect of a Short-Time Germination Process on the Nutrient Composition, Microbial Counts and Bread-Making Potential of Whole Flaxseed. J Food Proc Preserv. 2012

329 Fuller S and Stephens JM. Diosgenin, 4-hydroxyisoleucine, and fiber from fenugreek: mechanisms of actions and potential effects on metabolic syndrome. Adv Nutr. 2015

330 Amin A, Alkaabi A and Al-Falasi S. Chemopreventive activities of Trigonella foenum graecum (Fenugreek) against breast cancer. Cell Biol Int. 2005

331 Kaviarasan S, Ramamurty N and Gunasekaran P. Fenugreek (Trigonella Foenum Graecum) seed extract prevents ehanol-induced toxicity and apoptosis in changing liver cells. Alcohol Alcohol. 2006

332 Alsemari A, Alkhodairy F, Aldakan A, et al. The selective cytotoxic anti-cancer properties and proteomic analysis of Trigonella Foenum-Graecum. BMC Complement Altern Med. 2014

333 Al-Daghri NM, Alokail MS, Alkharfy KM, et al. Fenugreek extract as an inducer of cellular death via autophagy in human T lymphoma Jurkat cells. BMC Complement Altern Med. 2012

334 Nordeen SK, Bona BJ, Jones DN, et al. Endocrine disrupting activities of the flavonoid nutraceuticals luteolin and quercetin. Horm Cancer. 2013

335 Al-Yahya MA, Mossa JS, Ageel AM et al. Pharmacological and safety evaluation studies on Lepidium sativum L., Seeds. Phytomedicine. 1994

336 Maghrani M, Zeggwagh NA, Michel JB et al. Antihypertensive effect of Lepidium sativum L. in spontaneously hypertensive rats. J Ethnopharmacol. 2005

337 Najeeb-Ur-Rehman, Mehmood MH, Alkharfy KM, et al. Prokinetic and laxative activities of Lepidium sativum seed extract with species and tissue selective gut stimulatory actions. J Ethnopharmacol. 2011

338 Al-Sheddi ES, Farshori NN, Al-Oqail MM, et al. Protective effect of Lepidium sativum seed extract against hydrogen peroxide-induced cytotoxicity and oxidative stress in human liver cells (HepG2). Pharm Biol. 2016

339 Schmid D, Sacher R, Belser E, et al. Vegetable sprouts: a potent source for cosmetic actives. Naturals/Botanics. 2011

340 Regulation (EU) No 208/2013. The origin of the seeds has to be traceable always at all stages of processing, production and distribution. (see also Article 18 of Regulation (EC) No 178/2002)

341 Chaine A, Arnaud E, Kondjoyan A, et al. Effect of steam and lactic acid treatments on the survival of Salmonella Enteritidis and Campylobacter jejuni inoculated on chicken skin. Int J Food Microbiol. 2013

342 Martínez-Villaluenga C, Frías J, Gulewicz P, et al. Food safety evaluation of broccoli and radish sprouts. Food Chem Toxicol. 2008

343 Kintzel U. Red Clover in Sheep Pasture? *www.whitecloversheepfarm.com/prl-articles/FarmingMagazineRedCloverFall12.pdf*

344 Barnes S. Phyto-estrogens and osteoporosis: what is a safe dose? Br J Nutr. 2003

345 Lethaby A, Marjoribanks J, Kronenberg F, et al. Phytestrogens for menopausal vasomotor symptoms. Cochrane Database Syst Rev. 2013

346 Shapiro TA, Fahey JW, Dinkova-Kostova AT, et al Safety, tolerance, and metabolism of broccoli sprout glucosinolates and isothiocyanates: a clinical phase I study. Nutr Cancer. 2006

347 Pasko P, Bukowska-Strakova K, Gdula-Argasinska J, et al. Rutabaga (Brassica napus L. var. napobrassica) seeds, roots, and sprouts: a novel kind of food with antioxidant properties and proapoptotic potential in Hep G2 hepatoma cell line. J Med Food. 2013

348 Masci A, Mattioli R, Costantino P, et al. Neuroprotective Effect of Brassica oleracea Sprouts Crude Juice in a Cellular Model of Alzheimer's Disease. Oxidative Medicine and Cellular Longevity. 2015

349 McEwen DC. Ovarian failure and the Menopause. Can Med Assoc J. 1965

350   Castallo MA. Modern management of the menopause; this deficiency disease, caused by lack of ovarian hormone, should be treated throughout life by estrogen replacement therapy Pa Med. 1967

351   Armitage M, Nooney J and Stephen Evans. Recent concerns surrounding HRT. Clin Endocrinol (Oxf). 2003

352   Million Women Study Collaborators. Patterns of use of hormone replacement therapy in one million women in Britain, 1996-2000. BJOG. 2002

353   Vickers MR, Martin J, Meade TW, et al. Women's international study of long-duration estrogen after menopause (WISDOM): a randomised controlled trial. BMC Womens Health. 2007

354   Langer RD, Manson JE and Allison MA. Have we come full circle - or moved forward? The Women's Health Initiative 10 years on. Climacteric. 2012.

355   Dr Alastair H MacLennan: Writing in cardiology magazine *Heart Wire* (2007)

356   Burger HG, MacLennan AH, Huang KE, et al. Evidence-based assessment of the impact of the WHI on women's health. Climacteric. 2012

357   Jones ME, Schoemaker MJ, Wright L, et al. Menopausal hormone therapy and breast cancer: what is the true size of the increased risk? Br J Cancer. 2016

358   British Medical Journal Patient Summaries. *www.bestpractice.bmj.com/best-practice/pdf/patient-summaries/en-gb/532536.pdf*

359   Cumming GP, Currie HD, Panay N, et al. Stopping hormone replacement therapy: were women ill advised? Menopause Int. 2011

360   "Your HRT Agony Aunt" *www.dailymail.co.uk/health/article-202318/Your-HRT-Agony-Aunt.html*

361   Tice JA, Ettinger B, Ensrud K, et al. Phytestrogen supplements for the treatment of hot flashes: the Isoflavone Clover Extract (ICE) Study: a randomized controlled trial. JAMA. 2003

362   Peñalvo JL, Adlercreutz H, Uehara M, et al. Lignan content of selected foods from Japan. J Agric Food Chem. 2008

363   Kronenberg F, and Fugh-Berman A. Complementary and alternative medicine for menopausal symptoms: a review of randomized, controlled trials. Ann Intern Med. 2002

364   Shutt DA. The effects of plant estrogens on animal reproduction. Endeavour. 1976

365   Webb CM, Hayward CS, Mason MJ, et al. Coronary vasomotor and blood flow responses to isoflavone-intact soya protein in subjects with coronary heart disease or risk factors for coronary heart disease. Clin Sci (Lond). 2008

366   Mangano KM, Hutchins-Wiese HL, Kenny AM, et l Soy proteins and isoflavones reduce interleukin-6 but not serum lipids in older women: a randomized controlled trial. Nutr Res. 2013

367   Niu K, Momma H, Kobayashi Y, et al. The traditional Japanese dietary pattern and longitudinal changes in cardiovascular disease risk factors in apparently healthy Japanese adults. Eur J Nutr. 2016

368 Padhi EM, Blewett HJ, Duncan AM, et al. Whole Soy Flour Incorporated into a Muffin and Consumed at 2 Doses of Soy Protein Does Not Lower LDL Cholesterol in a Randomized, Double-Blind Controlled Trial of Hypercholesterolemic Adults. J Nutr. 2015

369 Ma D, Qin L, Liu B, et al. Inhibition of soy isoflavone intake on bone loss in menopausal women: evaluated by meta-analysis of randomized controlled trials. Wei Sheng Yan Jiu. 2009

370 Pawlowski JW, Martin BR, McCabe GP, et al. Impact of equol-producing capacity and soy-isoflavone profiles of supplements on bone calcium retention in postmenopausal women: a randomized crossover trial. Am J Clin Nutr. 2015

371 Occhiuto F, Pasquale RD, Guglielmo G, et al. Effects of phytestrogenic isoflavones from red clover (Trifolium pratense L.) on experimental osteoporosis. Phytother Res. 2007

372 Kawakita S, Marotta F, Naito Y, et al. Effect of an isoflavones-containing red clover preparation and alkaline supplementation on bone metabolism in ovariectomized rats. Clin Interv Aging. 2009

373 Shakeri F, Taavoni S, Goushegir A, Haghani H. Effectiveness of red clover in alleviating menopausal symptoms: a 12-week randomized, controlled trial. Climacteric. 2015

374 Pfitscher A, Reiter E, Jungbauer A. Receptor binding and transactivation activities of red clover isoflavones and their metabolites. J Steroid Biochem Mol Biol. 2008

375 Setchell KD, Brown NM and Lydeking-Olsen E. The clinical importance of the metabolite equol-a clue to the effectiveness of soy and its isoflavones. J Nutr. 2002

376 Mucci M, Carraro C, Mancino P, Monti M, Papadia LS, Volpini G, Benvenuti C. Soy isoflavones, lactobacilli, Magnolia bark extract, vitamin D3 and calcium. Controlled clinical study in menopause. Minerva Ginecol. 2006

377 Nagino T, Kano M, Masuoka N, et al. Intake of a fermented soymilk beverage containing moderate levels of isoflavone aglycones enhances bioavailability of isoflavones in healthy premenopausal Japanese women: a double-blind, placebo-controlled, single-dose, crossover trial. Biosci Microbiota Food Health. 2016

378 Xie B, Zhang S, Liu J, et al. Enhanced Estrogenic Activity of Soybean Isoflavones by Coadministration of Liuwei Dihuang Pills in Ovariectomized Rats. Phytother Res. 2015

379 Harvard Medical School have produced a nice summary of the debate. You can see it on *www.health.harvard.edu/womens-health/bioidentical-hormones-help-or-hype*

380 Stephenson K, Neuenschwander PF and Kurdowska AK. The effects of compounded bioidentical transdermal hormone therapy on hemostatic, inflammatory, immune factors; cardiovascular biomarkers; quality-of-life measures; and health outcomes in perimenopausal and postmenopausal women. Int J Pharm Compd. 2013

381   Ruiz AD and Daniels KR. The effectiveness of sublingual and topical compounded bioidentical hormone replacement therapy in postmenopausal women: an observational cohort study. Int J Pharm Compd. 2014

382   Pinkerton JVand Santoro N. Compounded bioidentical hormone therapy: identifying use trends and knowledge gaps among US women. Menopause. 2015

383   BBC Radio 4. *You and Yours*, first broadcast 13th July 2016

384   Craig ZR, Wang W and Flaws JA. Endocrine-disrupting chemicals in ovarian function: effects on steroidogenesis, metabolism and nuclear receptor signaling. Reproduction. 2011

385   Mlynarcikova A, Fickova M and Scsukova S. Impact of endocrine disruptors on ovarian steroidogenesis. Endocr Regul. 2014

386   Marques-Pinto A and Carvalho D. Human infertility: are endocrine disruptors to blame? Endocr Connect. 2013

387   Uzumcu M1, Zama AM and Oruc E. Epigenetic mechanisms in the actions of endocrine-disrupting chemicals: gonadal effects and role in female reproduction. Reprod Domest Anim. 2012

388   Zama AM and Uzumcu M.Front. Epigenetic effects of endocrine-disrupting chemicals on female reproduction: an ovarian perspective. Neuroendocrinol. 2010

389   Diamanti-Kandarakis E, Bourguignon JP, Giudice LC, Hauser R, Prins GS, Soto AM, Zoeller RT, Gore AC. Endocrine-disrupting chemicals: an Endocrine Society scientific statement. Endocr Rev. 2009

390   *http://e.hormone.tulane.edu/learning/docking-receptor-binding.html*

391   Lamb JC, Boffetta P, Foster WG, et al. Critical comments on the WHO-UNEP State of the Science of Endocrine Disrupting Chemicals - 2012. (2014) Regul Toxicol Pharmacol. 2014

392   Reardon, S. *Other primates share human taste for plant estrogens*. New Scientist. 11th April 2012.

393   Ansari R, Hughes C and Husain K. Ligand-Mediated Toxicology: Characterisation and Translational Prospects 2016 In book: *Translational Toxicology: Defining a New Therapeutic Discipline*, Chapter: 4, Publisher: Molecular and Integrative Toxicology, Springer International Publishing, Switzerland, Editors: Claude Hughes and Michael D. Waters, pp.113-137.

394   Hughes C and Tansey G. Phytestrogens and Reproductive Medicine. The Reproductive and developmental toxicology. Ed. Korach KS Marcel Dekker Inc. New York 1998 Page 278

395   Edocr Rev. Diamanti-Kandarakis E, Bourguignon JP, Giudice LC, et al. Endocrine-disrupting chemicals: an Endocrine Society scientific statement. 2009

396   Zoeller RT, Brown TR, Doan LL, et al. Endocrine-disrupting chemicals and public health protection: a statement of principles from the endocrine society. Endocrinology. 2012

397 Bergman Å, Becher G, Blumberg B, et al. Manufacturing doubt about endocrine disrupter science - A rebuttal of industry-sponsored critical comments on the UNEP/WHO report "State of the Science of Endocrine Disrupting Chemicals 2012". Regul Toxicol Pharmacol. 2015

398 Schwartza H, Sontaga G, Plumbb J. Inventory of phytestrogen databases. Food Chem. 2009

399 Kuhnlea GGC, Dell'Aquilaa C, Aspinalla SM, et al. Phytestrogen content of fruits and vegetables commonly consumed in the UK based on LC–MS and 13C-labelled standards. Food Chem. 2009

400 Hloucalová P, Skládanka J, Horký P, et al. Determination of Phytestrogen Content in Fresh-Cut Legume Forage. Animals (Basel). 2016

401 Huang M-H, Norris J, Han W, et al. Development of an updated phytestrogen database for use with the SWAN Food Frequency Questionnaire: intakes and food sources in a community-based, multiethnic cohort study. Nutr Cancer. 2012

402 Chung-Ja J, and Vasantha Rupasinghe H. Tables of Isoflavone, Coumestrol, and Lignan Data. In *Phytestrogens and Health*. Eds.Anderson J.J.B Sarwar Gilani G. AOCS Publishing, 2002.

403 Priyanjali Dixit, Saroj Ghaskadbi, Hari Mohan, et al. Antioxidant properties of germinated fenugreek seeds. Phytother Res. 2005

404 Ponce MA, Scervino JM, Erra-Balsells R, et al. Flavonoids from shoots, roots and roots exudates of Brassica alba. Phytochem. 2004

405 Oszmiański J. Kolniak-Ostek J and Wojdyło A. Application of ultra performance liquid chromatography-photodiode detector-quadrupole/time of flight-mass spectrometry (UPLC-PDA-Q/TOF-MS) method for the characterization of phenolic compounds of Lepidium sativum L. sprouts. E Food ResTech. 2013

406 Tundis R, Marrelli M, Conforti F, et al. Trifolium pratense and T. repens (Leguminosae): edible flower extracts as functional ingredients. Foods. 2015

407 Miean KH and Mohamed S. Flavonoid (Myricetin, Quercetin, Kaempferol, Luteolin, and Apigenin) Content of Edible Tropical Plants. J. Agric. Food Chem. 2001

408 Zheng W and Wang SY. Antioxidant activity and phenolic compounds in selected herbs. Journal of Agricultural and Food Chemistry 2001

409 Shan B, Cai YZ, Sun M, et al. Antioxidant capacity of 26 spice extracts and characterization of their phenolic constituents. Journal of Agricultural and Food Chemistry. 2005

410 Stewart A.J, Mullen W and Crozier A. 2000 Occurrence of flavonols in tomatoes and tomato-based products. Journal of Agricultural and Food Chemistry. 2000

Also of interest from Findhorn Press

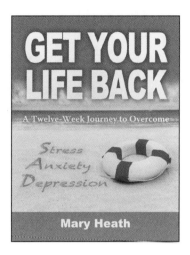

Get Your Life Back
A Twelve-Week Journey to Overcome
Stress – Anxiety – Depression
by Mary Heath

WITH MORE AND MORE DEMANDS AT WORK and in the home, the pace of life has become much faster over the past few decades. Increasingly, people struggle to fulfill all the expectations they are faced with, and start feeling stressed, anxious or depressed, sometimes to the point of burnout or breakdown.

If you are looking to step out of the stress cycle, regain your balance and get your life back, this tailored 12-week programme offers great support along the way. Each day presents you with relaxation, reflections and exercises to facilitate a positive change in your life. You will build your awareness with mindfulness, gain a better understanding on what causes stress and how to handle it, and find solutions for managing anxiety and panic attacks, for boosting your self-esteem and directions for the future. Relaxation and breathing exercises help to relax and control negative emotions; meditation, visualization and affirmations promote calm and reconnect you with your essence; yoga and other exercises support your body and mind; and practical tools such as goal setting and prioritizing assist you in organizing your life in a way that really serves you.

978-1-84409-677-0

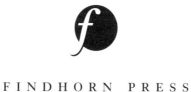

FINDHORN PRESS

Life-Changing Books

Consult our catalogue online
(with secure order facility) on
www.findhornpress.com

For information on the Findhorn Foundation:
www.findhorn.org